TRANSFORMING RACIAL AND CULTURAL LINES IN HEALTH AND SOCIAL CARE

This book proposes an innovative new model for transforming racial and cultural lines in health and social care through communication processes, and introduces listening partnerships as a cost-effective, sustainable intervention to improve communication skills.

Transforming Racial and Cultural Lines in Health and Social Care walks the reader through the process of developing the essential skills for racially and culturally effective and compassionate communication. Divided into four parts, the book includes examples that highlight the significance of each skill and provides listening partnerships on each topic. In the final part of the book, Froehlich and Thornton-Marsh interview medical, health, and social care practitioners regarding their experiences in using racially and culturally effective communication to transform health and social care. Improved communication enhances the experience of health and social care for both patients and practitioners and ultimately supports better health outcomes.

Transforming Racial and Cultural Lines in Health and Social Care is essential reading for health and social care students looking to improve their communication skills and provide better care.

Jan Froehlich is Associate Professor of Occupational Therapy at the University of New England (UNE), Maine, United States.

June Thornton-Marsh is a Licensed Clinical Social Worker in private practice, Maine, United States.

TRANSFORMING RACIAL AND CULTURAL LINES IN HEALTH AND SOCIAL CARE

Listening, Loving, and Lifting Spirits When You Can

Jan Froehlich and June Thornton-Marsh

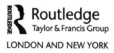

Routledge
Taylor & Francis Group

LONDON AND NEW YORK

First published 2021
by Routledge
2 Park Square, Milton Park, Abingdon, Oxon OX14 4RN

and by Routledge
52 Vanderbilt Avenue, New York, NY 10017

Routledge is an imprint of the Taylor & Francis Group, an informa business

British Library Cataloguing-in-Publication Data
A catalogue record for this book is available from the British Library

Library of Congress Cataloging-in-Publication Data
Names: Froehlich, Jan, author. | Thornton-Marsh, June, author.
Title: Transforming racial and cultural lines in health and social care: listening,
loving, and lifting spirits when you can / Jan Froehlich and June Thornton-Marsh.
Description: Abingdon, Oxon ; New York, NY : Routledge, 2021. |
Includes bibliographical references and index.
Identifiers: LCCN 2020035774 (print) | LCCN 2020035775 (ebook) |
ISBN 9780367259037 (hbk) | ISBN 9780367258993 (pbk) |
ISBN 9780429290466 (ebk)
Subjects: LCSH: Intercultural communication. |
Social work administration. | Medical care.
Classification: LCC HM1211 .F75 2021 (print) |
LCC HM1211 (ebook) | DDC 303.48/2–dc23
LC record available at https://lccn.loc.gov/2020035774
LC ebook record available at https://lccn.loc.gov/2020035775

ISBN: 978-0-367-25903-7 (hbk)
ISBN: 978-0-367-25899-3 (pbk)
ISBN: 978-0-429-29046-6 (ebk)

Typeset in Bembo
by Newgen Publishing UK

Art by Kiri Guyaz

We dedicate this book to health and social care practitioners across the globe who have committed their life work to improving the health and the wellbeing of clients, communities, and populations on this planet. We acknowledge the many members of health and social care teams who sacrifice their lives while fulfilling their calling to serve others. We call for a radical transformation in systems of health and social care delivery that ask frontline workers to put themselves unnecessarily in harm's way. We will not forget your sacrifices!

En Solidaridad,
Jan and June

CONTENTS

FIGURES

TABLES

VIGNETTES

PREFACE

About June

From an early age, I recognized human resilience in the midst of human suffering. My mother was an immigrant Japanese woman who embodied her ancestral Samurai spirit when she left Japan in the wake of the suffering inflicted by the atomic bombs. My father embodied the strength and dignity instilled by his tribal kin – African ancestors who survived their enslavement and indigenous forebearers who survived genocide. I became skilled in seeing the light in others and in myself and ultimately was drawn to a community of like-hearted social workers committed to uplifting the human spirit while lessening human suffering.

Years later, as a social worker in a predominantly white organization, in an overwhelmingly white state, I struggled to find the depth of authentic human connection and the synergistic life force with others that I needed to thrive. I had begun to notice increasing anger, bone-numbing exhaustion, and a deafening hopelessness building within me. Without a community of spirited and collaborative allies, I suffered. I found an unexpected ally in Jan, a white occupational therapist. As I shared stories of pain honed from experiences of isolation, racism, and rejection, Jan listened with love, compassion, and hopefulness. Missing was the denial, guilt, shame, helplessness, or shock that I was familiar with when sharing those types of experiences with white people. In ever-increasing collaborative exchanges, we were both transformed. I found with Jan a most powerful partner for life – a co-conspirator committed to transforming pain and suffering into healing and flourishing.

About Jan

As a young white female of Irish, German, and Scottish heritage, I was inspired by the kindness, generosity, and humour in my mixed Catholic/Protestant white family and friends. Yet I also saw harshness, pain, disconnection, and the pull to addictions. Racism, sexism, and classism also reared their ugly heads and left me indignant. I felt particularly pained by racism and felt lost about how to inter-rupt it. Catholicism connected me with an awareness of the pain and suffering in the global human family and offered me hope and community in the fight for a better world for all people. Fortunately, when I discovered occupational therapy, my chosen profession became an additional vehicle for social change. Joining with occupational therapists and other health professionals to fight for better lives for all people – particularly for people with disabilities, people with mental health labels, and for all oppressed people – became a richly rewarding journey and deeply meaningful occupation.

On this journey, I found that building open, honest, and loving friendships with people from all backgrounds, but particularly with Black and Indigenous people, profoundly changed my life. They corrected me when I made mistakes, teased me about my whiteness, held out that I and other white people were good, and that we needed much healing from the damage of racism. Over time, they opened up about the hurts of multiple oppressions in their lives. When I met June, I felt an immediate kinship between us. She was as determined as I was to take action to end racism and all forms of oppression in the world and to place connection and enjoyment at the centre of that work.

About our journey of transforming racial and cultural lines

Over time, we shared the painful experiences of oppression in our lives. Racial and cultural divisions between us dissolved into tears and laughter as we listened, loved, and lifted spirits with each other. We became committed to sharing this process with other health and social care practitioners. Out of our relationship, we gave birth to our book, *Transforming Racial and Cultural Lines in Health and Social Care: Listening, Loving, and Lifting Spirits When You Can.*

The goal of this unique interprofessional book on racially and culturally effective communication is to facilitate the development of effective communica-tion within and across racial and cultural lines as a mechanism for transforming the many divisions that limit progress in health and social care. Improved communica-tion within and across racial and cultural lines enhances the experience of health and social care for clients as well as for members of health and social care teams, and ultimately supports better health outcomes. We envision that many health and social care students and practitioners will find our book relevant; it is an important book for people of all backgrounds across the world. Throughout the book, we interchangeably refer to practitioners either by their full designations or by their abbreviations to reflect the reality of how members of health and social care teams address each other (for practitioner abbreviations, see Table 0.1). We acknowledge that the practitioners addressed in our book represent only several of the dozens of types of health and social care practitioner who contribute to the health and well-being of all people. We acknowledge and honour them as well as the practitioners addressed in our book for their essential work.

TABLE 0.1 Practitioner abbreviations

Certified Nurse Assistant	CNA
Nurse	RN
Nurse Practitioner	NP
Occupational Therapist	OT
Physical Therapist	PT
Physician	MD
Physician Assistant	PA
Social Worker	MSW or BSW

Most of us were called to be health and social care practitioners to promote the health and wellbeing of the bodies, hearts, and souls of human beings who need our compassionate presence. We have a deep awareness of the recovery that is possible when we use our minds and our hearts to ease the emotional, physical, and spiritual suffering of others. Despite our call to heal, many of us are "careworn" by the pressures of time and productivity within health and social care systems. This is especially true in frontline battles against pandemics, epidemics, plagues, and their aftermath. We challenge discouragement and compassion fatigue in the face of the deprivation, trauma, and complex needs of clients, patients, and colleagues as we reach for life, optimal health, and optimal wellbeing. We fight the threats to health and wellbeing experienced by racial and cultural identity groups. Our successes are multiplied when we join forces with our clients and all members of the health and social care teams. We know what is possible from deep loving kindness and connections when an interprofessional team can listen, love, and lift spirits not only with our clients but with each other. Though the body, soul, and mind can harness the healing generated from this collaboration, we acknowledge that it can often be extremely difficult to find within us the chutzpah and skill to listen, love, and lift spirits. Yet we can.

Part I: One human race with a tapestry of cultures: A communication process for transforming racial and cultural lines in health and social care

Fostering caring communication and connections within and across racial and cultural lines is at the heart of our book. In Part I, the authors highlight the reality that there is only one human race, and within that race, there are many rich and varied cultures. The myth of race is exposed as a social construct invented for the purposes of justifying the economic exploitation of groups of people using insignificant human differences, i.e. skin colour, as a pretext. A model for transforming racial and cultural lines in health and social care through a communication process is proposed. Listening partnerships, a confidential exchange of listening, are introduced as a cost-effective, sustainable intervention to improve communication skills. Case vignettes are introduced in this part of the book. They provide rich examples of relationships transforming racial and cultural lines in health and social care.

Additional components of the model that are fostered by listening partnerships include deepening awareness of self and others; skill development in listening, loving, and lifting spirits; deepening connections within and across racial and cultural lines; and an emphasis on action as inherent and designated leaders transforming health and wellbeing for humans and the planet. The Froehlich Communication Survey, the Treasuring the Human Race Survey, and the Racial and Cultural Awareness and Action Survey (see Appendix B) are introduced to increase awareness of strengths, areas for improvement, and goals related to racially and culturally effective communication. In addition, a Treasuring All Life Survey deepens awareness of the interrelationship between the health and wellbeing of all humans and the health of the planet and supports action steps (see Appendix B).

Part II: Refinement of racially and culturally effective communication in health care

In Part II, the reader is walked through the process of developing the specific skills necessary to listen, love, and lift spirits across and within racial and cultural lines. Each chapter addresses particular skills including presence and attunement, loving and inviting, lifting spirits, aligning and responding, and teamwork in health care. Most of the case vignettes are included in this part of the book to provide the reader with specific examples of racially and culturally effective communication. The exquisite diversity of languages spoken by clients is also illustrated to foster awareness of culturally and linguistically appropriate care. As in all communication, translations may not capture the exact nuances of what was expressed. Reflecting the realities of practice in health and social care both with and without physical distancing, practitioner examples include experiences before, during, and as a result of the coronavirus pandemic that began in 2019. Listening partnerships on each topic are facilitated in this part of the book to enhance skill development. Tables at the end of each chapter, also consolidated in Appendix C, provide listening partnership and journal prompts to support connection and skill development.

Part III: Deepening connections within and across racial and cultural lines

Part III introduces the concepts of oppression and internalized oppression and facilitates the process of dismantling oppression through engaged listening. The sociocultural determinants of health, as well as the impact of environmental exposures on the health of individuals, populations, and communities, are also addressed and further developed in Appendix D ("Health and wellbeing of people under threat"), with particular attention paid to the effect of the coronavirus pandemic on vulnerable groups. Additional topics for listening partnerships, discussion, and journalling, as well as practitioner examples, address the complexities of deepening connections within and across racial and cultural lines. The process of listening and being listened to is further developed to transform relationships across and within racial and cultural lines.

Part IV: Garnering love, hope, and leadership for human and planetary health

In Part IV, a variety of health professionals from diverse racial and cultural backgrounds, some interviewed prior to the coronavirus pandemic and some interviewed in the midst of the pandemic, share what they are most proud of in relation to their profession and the challenges they face. Experiences with listening, loving, and lifting spirits within and across racial and cultural lines are highlighted. Leadership experiences, the interrelationship between human and planetary health and wellbeing, and visions for health and social care systems that support the flourishing of all racial and cultural groups are explored.

Part IV also addresses the complex realities of jobs in health and social care – job satisfaction, compassion satisfaction, compassion fatigue, and burnout. The Quadruple Aim, which comprises improving health outcomes, decreasing costs, improving the experience of care for patients or clients, and for the practitioner is explored. The significance of both inherent leadership and designated leadership in improving experiences in health and social care for both clients and practitioners is highlighted. Our model, Leadership for Transforming Racial and Cultural Lines in Health and Social Care, identifies the principles and actionable skills necessary to inspire, lead, and organize health and social care teams to listen, love, and lift spirits. Enactment of this model holds the promise of improving health and wellbeing for all.

ACKNOWLEDGEMENTS

Our interviewees

We acknowledge the following interviewees who exemplify the heart and soul of health and social care practitioners. Their voices are expressed in Chapter 11: "Hopes and visions for human and planetary health: Voices of frontline workers as leaders".

Bill Wong, OTD, Adjunct Faculty, Stanbridge University, Monterey Park, CA, OT Practitioner at Interface Rehab, Placentia, California, United States.

Carl Toney, PA, Health Care Planning Consultant/Charter Member and Past President, Association of Clinicians for the Underserved (ACU), Scarborough, Maine, United States.

Islane Louis, BSN, MSN, RN, Nurse at the University of Vermont Health Network, Clinical Instructor, University of Vermont, Chittenden County, Vermont, United States.

Joshua Pastor, MS, OTR/L, Rogue Pediatric Therapies, Medford, OR, United States.

Kelli Fox, MSW, LCSW, CCS, LADC, Associate Program Director, Director of BSW Field Education, University of New England School of Social Work, Biddeford and Portland, Maine, United States.

Marie Roy, MSW, OTR/L, Hospice Social Worker, Hospice of Southern Maine, Scarborough, Maine, United States.

Patricia Rhodes, BS, OTR/L, has worked in a variety of rehabilitation facilities but is currently unemployed due to cutbacks during the coronavirus pandemic, Woodbury, Minnesota, United States.

Regina Phillips, BA, MSW, Grants and Community Engagement Coordinator, Westbrook School Department, Westbrook, Maine; and

Adjunct Faculty, University of New England School of Social Work, Portland, Maine, United States.

Sabine Diasonama, Cultural Broker, Maine Immigrant Rights Coalition, Portland, Maine, United States.

Said Nafai, OTD, MS, OTR/L, CLT, Assistant Professor of Occupational Therapy, American International College, Springfield, Massachusetts, United States.

Saige Purser, BA, Nikan'usk Manager, Youth Engagement Manager, Wabanaki Public Health, Bangor, Maine, United States.

Steve Kim, PT, DPT, CPA (inactive), Therapist, AFFIRMA Rehabilitation in Los Altos, California; and Freelance Therapist, ANX Home Health Care and Hospice Care, San Jose, California, United States.

Usha Reddi, MD, Pulmonologist, Olympic Memorial Hospital, Port Angeles, Washington, United States.

Our family and friends

We acknowledge our family and friends for their support and the unconditional love they have generously given to us throughout the process of birthing this transformational book. They have taught us how to listen, to love, and to lift sprits. June acknowledges Charles Thornton, Nobo Thornton, Michael Thornton, Madi Vannaman, Margie Thornton, and Dylan Marsh. Jan acknowledges Jeanette and Robert Froehlich, Michael and Marlena Hatem, Carolyn Mellone, and Marie Roy. June and Jan both acknowledge leaders in the International Re-evaluation Counseling Communities and the National Coalition Building Institute (NCBI) as key mentors.

Routledge

We acknowledge the entire staff at Routledge for their impeccable talent in co-creating with us. In particular, we acknowledge Grace McInnes, senior editor, for her pivotal editorial advice in planting the seeds for the direction of our manuscript and Evie Lonsdale, our editorial assistant, for her guidance in polishing a book we are proud of.

Newgen

We acknowledge Helen Lund, copy-editor, and Kelly Winter, project manager, for their phenomenal attention to detail and for patiently guiding our book toward perfection.

PART I

One human race with a tapestry of cultures

A communication process for transforming racial and cultural lines in health and social care

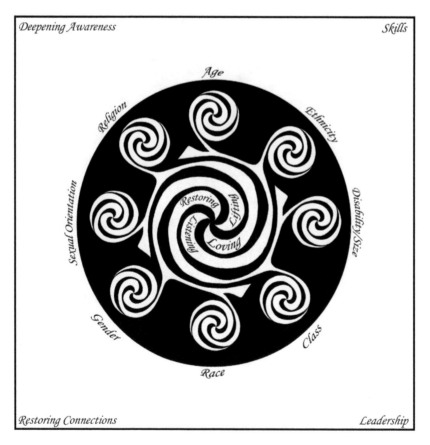

FIGURE 1.1 A model for transforming racial and cultural lines in health and social care

PART I MODEL COMPONENTS
INTRODUCTION TO LISTENING PARTNERSHIPS WITHIN AND ACROSS RACIAL AND CULTURAL LINES IN HEALTH AND SOCIAL CARE

Deepening awareness (surveys, experiences, reflection)

- Awareness of self
- Awareness of others
- Awareness of self with others
- Awareness of others' awareness of you
- Awareness of all living things

1

THE ART OF RACIALLY AND CULTURALLY EFFECTIVE COMMUNICATION IN HEALTH AND SOCIAL CARE

One human race with a tapestry of cultures

Humans are a remarkable species – more alike than different in our depth of caring and intelligent nature. In fact, we are 99.9% identical in genetic make-up. (National Human Genome Research Institute, 2018). Despite our similarities, we are often divided by racial and cultural lines, and these divisions limit our endeavours for a better world, particularly a world with transformative health and wellbeing as our birthright. There is only one race – the human race with a rich multilayered tapestry of varied and beautiful cultures. Race has been used as an artificial construct invented and used as a vicious tool to justify the economic exploitation of groups of people based on insignificant differences – i.e. skin colour. It's a minor presence in 500 of the 200,000 years modern humans have inhabited our planet (a mere 0.25% of human existence), and the unwavering commitment humans have made towards ending racism in the past 65 years (beginning with Rosa Parks refusing to give up her seat to a white man), spells its eventual and inevitable doom. Yet persistent and indefatigable engagements to transform racial and cultural lines must continue in order to undo the tremendous misunderstanding, miscommunication, and damage that continues to occur along these lines and bring about a better world for all humans.

Cultural lines also often differentiate and separate groups of people from the inherent connections we have with each other. Culture generally refers to "the ways of life" of a particular people – their ordinary and extraordinary behaviour, habits, values, and language(s). Parallel to the distinct culture of various ethnic groups, identity groups related to race, gender, socioeconomic class, age, sexual orientation, religion, and disability also have their own shared values, experiences, and "ways of being" that can be described as cultural. Similarly, occupational groups, such as doctors, nurses, factory workers, teachers, etc. tend to share norms and social behaviours that comprise a distinct culture, "ways of being" or "ways of life".

While all racial, cultural, and identity groups have many cherished strengths and positive attributes that are to be empowered, promoted, and celebrated, these groups also experience numerous challenges in contemporary society – many of which stem from their systematic and methodical mistreatment as members of their particular racial and cultural groups. Human suffering, shortened lives, and loss of lives from the health consequences of mistreatment along racial and cultural lines are well documented in the literature on health disparities and social determinants of health (SDH). Fortunately, the transformation of racial and cultural lines in society and in health care is gaining momentum as humans reach for each other, and as we struggle to create not only equitable health and social care systems, but a just world made possible as we deconstruct those lines. This transformation is fuelled by human caring, intelligence, courage, collaboration, and action that find nourishment in the deepening of human connections within and across racial and cultural lines. It is possible to further harness and accelerate this momentum by a skilful and profound communication process that embraces a particular way of listening, loving, and lifting spirits.

The nature of human communication

Communication is a means of connecting humans that involves the complex exchange of verbal and non-verbal information, experiences, and emotions. At its best, communication is aware, accurate, loving, creative, artful, and engaged – information, listening, and caring are exchanged as people reveal themselves to one another. Deep and loving connections within and across racial and cultural groups are forged on the battleground of insignificant differences. Creativity and healing are often generated from those spaces where humans choose to meet in a place of possibility. Because human communication is so complex, there is enormous potential for deep healing connections, deep understanding, and flexibility as both speaker and listener transform. However, miscommunications, mistakes, conflict, painful emotions, and rigid formulations can also easily occur as people attempt to share information, experiences, and connections with one another, especially across, but also within racial and cultural lines. The good news is that it isn't difficult for most people to be taught and to learn how to be more effective and transformative communicators. This is a requisite for best practice in health and social care.

The significance of effective communication in health and social care

There is a growing body of research which shows that kindness, compassion, listening, and connecting have a profound effect on healing (Doty, 2016; Trzeciak et al., 2019). While a compassionate and open bedside manner was historically considered less important than a health practitioner's technical skills, the significance of effective communication and its impact on the quality of care are now cited across health and social care literature (Alpert, 2011; Boschma et al., 2010;

Davis & Musolino, 2016; Joint Commission, 2015; Lingard et al., 2008; Kohn et al., 2000; Merlino, 2017; Sargeant et al., 2011; Taylor, 2008). Multiple studies show that kindness, caring, and effective communication between practitioners and patients or clients actually improve health and wellness outcomes (Griffin et al., 2004; Kelley et al., 2014; Miller et al., 2005; Rakel et al., 2009; Street et al., 2009; Wampold & Brown, 2005). Additionally, ineffective communication is identified as one of the leading causes of medical errors (Kern, 2016; Leonard et al., 2004; Lingard et al., 2008; Sutcliffe et al., 2004; Woolf et al., 2004). Medical errors are the third leading cause of death in the United States (Makary & Daniel, 2016).

Cultural competence, multicultural competence, and racial-cultural competence and effectiveness

According to the U.S. Department of Health and Human Services (USDHHS), cultural competence

> refers to the ability to honor and respect the beliefs, languages, interpersonal styles, and behaviors of individuals and families receiving services, as well as staff members who are providing such services. Cultural competence is a dynamic, ongoing developmental process that requires a long-term commitment and is achieved over time.
>
> *USDHHS, 2003, p. 12*

Not surprisingly, a significant body of literature identifies cultural competence as an important factor that improves communication and collaboration, increases client and practitioner satisfaction, enhances adherence to health recommendations, improves outcomes and reduces health disparities, while also highlighting the need for ongoing improvement and measurement of our efforts (Betancourt et al., 2014; Clifford et al., 2015; Committee on Pediatric Workforce, American Academy of Pediatrics, 2004; Kripalani et al., 2006; Minnican & O'Toole, 2020; Ulrey & Amason, 2001).

There are several concepts closely related to cultural competence – racial-cultural competence, cultural effectiveness, and multicultural competence. For example, Sue and Torino (2005) highlighted the need to address not just cultural competence, but racial-cultural competence in counselling and therapy. Stone (2006) proposed that beyond cultural competence, cultural effectiveness is "the ability to interact with people from different cultures so as to optimize the probability of mutually successful outcomes" (p. 338). Kivel (2007) noted that white cultural dominance is embedded in efforts to enhance cultural competence. Therefore, he advocated for multicultural competence or genuine fluency in more than one culture. As he eloquently stated,

> Part of being multiculturally competent is realizing the limits of your understanding. It should make you less arrogant and more humble. It should

provide you with skills for promoting the leadership of those from the cultures in which you are competent. As we become more multiculturally competent, we increase our effectiveness in working with diverse populations, but we cannot substitute for people who are experts in their own culture.

Kivel, 2007, p. 4

Models and frameworks for cultural competence and effectiveness

Although concepts, models, and frameworks related to racial-cultural and multicultural competence and effectiveness are evolving, a review of key concepts and current frameworks and models informs and advances efforts to transform racial and cultural lines in health and social care. As Dean (2001) proposed in her seminal article, "The Myth of Cross-Cultural Competence", cultural competence is not achievable because of the dynamic, ever-changing, and ever-evolving nature of culture. In other words, there is no endpoint in learning about different cultural groups because they are not static. One must continually be engaged in learning, adapting, and responding flexibly in interactions with people who are different from ourselves. Additionally, she invites practitioners to participate in the journey of actually appreciating one's own "cultural incompetence" while seeking to understand and build relationships in our cross-cultural work.

Many important models and frameworks for developing cultural competence and cultural effectiveness for practitioners capture the dynamic and relational nature of cultural interactions described by Dean (see Table 1.1). Campinha-Bacote (2007), a nationally and internationally recognized scholar and educational leader in the field of nursing, developed a process of cultural competence in the delivery of health care. Wells et al. (2016), scholars and leaders in the field of occupational therapy, describe a model for cultural effectiveness. Lattanzi, an educational leader in physical therapy collaborated with Purnell (Lattanzi & Purnell, 2006), another educational leader and scholar in the field of nursing, and developed steps to cultural study and cultural competence in physical therapy. Building upon Sue's earlier work (2001), Sue et al. (2016) developed a multidimensional model of cultural competence in social work.

Cultural awareness, cultural knowledge, and cultural skills

Each of the cultural competence or cultural effectiveness models highlighted in Table 1.1. has many distinct features, yet each shares an emphasis on the development of cultural self-awareness, increasing cultural knowledge, and developing cultural skills through an open, willing attitude and engagement in cross-cultural experiences. Self-exploration fosters increased awareness, sensitivity, and appreciation of one's own identity groups and is integral to the process of becoming increasingly aware, sensitive, and appreciative of other racial and cultural identities. Self-exploration also fosters racial and cultural humility by allowing one to

TABLE 1.1 Cultural competence models and frameworks in health and social care

Common goals across cultural competence models and frameworks	The Process of Cultural Competence in the Delivery of Healthcare Services (Nursing) (Campinha-Bacote, 2007)	Model for Cultural Effectiveness (Occupational Therapy) (Wells et al., 2016)	Lattanzi's Steps to Culturally Competent Practice for Physical Therapists (Lattanzi & Purnell, 2006)	Multidimensional Model of Cultural Competence in Social Work – Components of Cultural Competence (Sue et al., 2016)
Deepening cultural self-awareness	Deliberate exploration of one's heritage, biases, stereotypes, prejudices, assumptions, and "isms"	Self-exploration of one's own biases and one's cultural, racial, and ethnic heritage	Exploration of one's own cultural heritage and level of cultural competence	Active engagement in becoming aware of one's own values, biases, and assumptions about human behaviour
Increasing cultural knowledge	Cultural knowledge of health-related beliefs, practices, values, diseases, treatment, and interaction styles	Development of cultural knowledge and a deeper understanding of privilege, power, and the dynamics of oppression	Understanding primary (i.e. gender, race, age, etc.) and secondary (i.e. educational status, political beliefs, marital status, etc.) characteristics of culture	Active attempts to understand the worldview of culturally diverse clients
Developing cultural skills	Cultural skill in obtaining relevant cultural data, a cultural and spiritual assessment, and communicating with cultural sensitivity	Cultural skill development focuses on culturally and linguistically appropriate communication, assessments, and interventions	Successful cross-cultural interaction and communication skills are built upon identifying and respecting differences	Active development and practice of culturally appropriate, relevant, and sensitive communication, interventions, and techniques

(continued)

TABLE 1.1 (Cont.)

Common goals across cultural competence models and frameworks	The Process of Cultural Competence in the Delivery of Healthcare Services (Nursing) (Campinha-Bacote, 2007)	Model for Cultural Effectiveness (Occupational Therapy) (Wells et al., 2016)	Lattanzi's Steps to Culturally Competent Practice for Physical Therapists (Lattanzi & Purnell, 2006)	Multidimensional Model of Cultural Competence in Social Work – Components of Cultural Competence (Sue et al., 2016)
Unique goals and/or features				
	Cultural encounters are viewed as sacred opportunities to establish a therapeutic alliance with those who are different from us and are a must for health practitioners	Critical reflection both in action, on action, and for action to increase cultural effectiveness	Culturally congruent PT evaluations, short- and long-term goals, and interventions are identified and implemented	Understanding organizational and institutional forces that enhance or diminish cultural competence and implementing multicultural organizational development
	Cultural desire or genuine motivation to understand, appreciate, respect, and care for people who are different from ourselves is inspired and fostered	Consideration of and reflection upon the influence of contextual nuances to support cultural effectiveness	Cultural competence progression: unconscious incompetence to conscious incompetence to conscious competence to unconscious competence	Understanding group-specific worldviews of multiple identity groups is considered a component of cultural competence. Foci of cultural competence are at the clinical, professional, organizational, and societal levels of intervention

recognize that there is much we don't know or understand about racial and cultural groups who are different from ourselves, and that mistakes are inevitable as we reach to connect across racial and cultural lines. Mistakes become opportunities for reflection and growth. Increasing one's racial and cultural knowledge while also deepening one's understanding of privilege, power, and the dynamics of oppression supports practitioners in developing racial and cultural competence. Understanding important historical information and some generalities regarding racial and cultural groups, yet learning to respond flexibly to each unique individual, family, group, or community with awareness of each unique context is essential. Cultural skills support the provision of culturally responsive and relevant care and include conducting culturally appropriate assessments, providing culturally appropriate interventions, and communicating effectively within and across racial and cultural lines in interactions with clients, communities, peers, and colleagues.

Racially and culturally effective communication

Racially and culturally effective communication is at the core of racial-cultural competence and effectiveness. It is a vital key to delivering optimal care. Given the ever-present, conscious or unconscious dimensions of race and culture in human interactions, it seems apparent that any meaningful definition of effective communication must encompass the dimensions of race and culture. Reflecting an integration of key concepts previously cited regarding effective communication, racial-cultural competence, and effectiveness, we propose a working definition of effective communication as racially and culturally effective communication:

> *the artful interplay between listening, speaking, and caring coupled with awareness, sensitivity, appreciation, and responsiveness to verbal and non-verbal communication and emotions while welcoming racial and cultural diversity and supporting connection, understanding, and mutually successful outcomes.*

Communication that transforms racial and cultural lines

Racially and culturally effective communication honours the reality that we are not perfect communicators and invites the exquisitely human journey of making mistakes as we reach for one another within and across racial and cultural lines that divide individuals, groups, families, and communities. It does not ignore or blur racial and cultural differences, but advances deeper appreciation, restorative connections, and greater effectiveness within and across racial and cultural groups. Racially and culturally effective communication transforms the present lives of people and the future narrative of what is possible within individuals, families, groups, and communities. Creative, caring, and effective verbal and non-verbal communication requires a heart-driven practice with honest feedback, humility, and thoughtful reflection – ideally with individuals, groups, and communities from a wide array of racial and cultural backgrounds. It is only with courage, practice, a willingness to make mistakes, and supportive feedback that allows for clarity, effectiveness, flexibility, awareness, and understanding, that deeper loving connections emerge. A model for transforming racial and cultural lines, through a communication process that honours all, unfolds in the following chapters.

References

Alpert, J. (2011). Some simple rules for effective communication in clinical teaching and practice environments. *The American Journal of Medicine, 124*(5), 381–382. https://doi.org/10.1016/j.amjmed.2010.11.026

Betancourt, J. R., Corbett, J., & Bondaryk, M. R. (2014). Addressing disparities and achieving equity: Cultural competence, ethics, and health-care transformation. *Chest, 145*(1), 143–148. https://doi.org/10.1378/chest.13-0634

Boschma, G., Einboden, R., Groening, M., Jackson, C., MacPhee, M., Marshall, H., … Roberts, E. (2010). Strengthening communication education in an undergraduate nursing curriculum. *International Journal of Nursing Education Scholarship, 7*(1), 1–14. https://doi.org/10.2202/1548-923X.2043

Campinha-Bacote, J. (2007). *The process of cultural competence in the delivery of health care services: The journey continues* (5th ed.). Blue Ash, OH: Transcultural C.A.R.E. Associates.

Clifford, A., McCalman, J., Bainbridge, R., & Tsey, K. (2015). Interventions to improve cultural competency in health care for Indigenous peoples of Australia, New Zealand, Canada and the USA: A systematic review. *International Journal for Quality in Health Care, 27*(2), 89–98. https://doi.org/10.1093/intqhc/mzv010

Committee on Pediatric Workforce, American Academy of Pediatrics (2004). Ensuring culturally effective pediatric care: Implications for education and health policy. *Pediatrics, 114*(6), 1677–1685. https://doi.org/10.1542/peds.2004-2091

Davis, C. M., & Musolino, G. M. (2016). *Patient practitioner interaction* (6th ed.). Thorofare, NJ: SLACK, Inc.

Dean, R. G. (2001). The myth of cross-cultural competence. *Families in Society: The Journal of Contemporary Social Services, 82*(6), 623–630. https://doi.org/10.1606/1044-3894.151

Doty, J. R. (2016, January 26). The blog: Why kindness heals. *Huffington Post.* www.huffingtonpost.com/james-r-doty-md/why-kindness-heals_b_9082134.html

Griffin, S. J., Kinmonth, A. L., Veltman, M. W., Gillard, S., Grant, J., & Steward, M. (2004). Effect on health-related outcomes of interventions to alter the interaction between patients and practitioners: A systematic review of trials. *The Annals of Family Medicine, 2*(6), 595–608. https://doi.org/10.1370/afm.142

Joint Commission (2015). Sentinel event data: Root causes by event type. www.jointcommission.org/assets/1/23/jconline_April_29_15.pdf

Kelley, J. M., Kraft-Todd, G., Schapira, L., Kossowsky, J., & Riess, H. (2014). The influence of the patient-clinician relationship on healthcare outcomes: A systematic review and meta-analysis of randomized controlled trials. *PLoS ONE, 9*(4), e94207. https://doi.org/10.1371/journal.pone.0094207

Kern, C. (2016, February 11). Healthcare miscommunication costs 2,000 lives and $1.7 billion annually. Health IT Outcomes, News feature. www.healthitoutcomes.com/doc/healthcare-miscommunication-costs-lives-and-billion-0001

Kivel, P. (2007). Multicultural competence. http://paulkivel.com/wp-content/uploads/2015/07/multiculturalcompetence.pdf

Kohn, L. T., Corrigan, J., Donaldson, M. S., & Committee on Quality of Health Care in America, & Institute of Medicine (2000). *To err is human: Building a safer health system.*

Washington, DC: National Academy Press. (2nd ed. published 2010). https://doi.org/10.17226/9728

Kripalani, S., Bussey-Jones, J., Katz, M. G., & Genao, I. (2006). A prescription for cultural competence in medical education. *Journal of General Internal Medicine, 21*(10), 1116–1120. https://doi.org/10.1111/j.1525-1497.2006.00557.x

Lattanzi, J. B., & Purnell, L. D. (2006). *Developing cultural competence in physical therapy.* Philadelphia, PA: F.A. Davis Company.

Leonard, M., Graham, S., & Bonacum, D. (2004). The human factor: The critical importance of effective teamwork and communication in providing safe care. *Quality and Safety in Health Care, 13*(Suppl_1), i85–i90. https://doi.org/10.1136/qshc.2004.010033

Lingard, L., Regehr, G., Orser, B., Reznick, R., Baker, G. R., Doran, D., … White, S. (2008). Evaluation of a preoperative checklist and team briefing among surgeons, nurses, and anesthesiologists to reduce failures in communication. *Archives of Surgery, 143*(1), 12. https://doi.org/10.1001/archsurg.2007.21

Makary, M. A., & Daniel, M. (2016). Medical error: The third leading cause of death in the U.S. *British Medical Journal, 353*(i2139). https://doi.org/10.1136/bmj.i2139

Merlino, J. (2017, November 6). Communication: A critical healthcare competency. PSQH: Patient Safety & Quality Health Care. www.psqh.com/analysis/communication-critical-healthcare-competency/

Miller, S. D., Duncan, B. L., Sorrell, R., & Brown, G. S. (2005). The partners for change outcome management system. *Journal of Clinical Psychology, 61*(2), 199–208. https://doi.org/10.1002/jclp.20111

Minnican, C., & O'Toole, G. (2020). Exploring the incidence of culturally responsive communication in Australian healthcare: The first rapid review on this concept. *BMC Health Services Research, 20,* 1–14. https://doi.org/10.1186/s12913-019-4859-6

National Human Genome Research Institute (2018). Human genomic variation. NIH. www.genome.gov/dna-day/15-ways/human-genomic-variation

Rakel, D. P., Hoeft, T. J., Barrett, B. P., Chewning, B. A., Craig, B. M., & Niu, M. (2009). Practitioner empathy and the duration of the common cold. *Family Medicine, 41*(7), 494.

Sargeant, J., MacLeod, T., & Murray, A. (2011). An interprofessional approach to teaching communication skills. *Journal of Continuing Education in the Health Professions, 31*(4), 265–267. https://doi.org/10.1002/chp.20139

Stone, N. (2006). Conceptualizing intercultural effectiveness for university teaching. *Journal of Studies in International Education, 10,* 334–356. http://dx.doi.org/10.1177/1028315306287634

Street, R. L., Makoul, G., Arora, N. K., & Epstein, R. M. (2009). How does communication heal? Pathways linking clinician–patient communication to health outcomes. *Patient Education and Counseling, 74*(3), 295–301. https://doi.org/10.1016/j.pec.2008.11.015

Sue, D. W. (2001). Multidimensional facets of cultural competence. *The Counseling Psychologist, 29*(6), 790–821. https://doi.org/10.1177/0011000001296002

Sue, D. W., Rasheed, J. M., & Rasheed, M. N. (2016). *Multicultural social work practice: A competency-based approach to diversity and social justice.* Hoboken, NJ: Jossey-Bass. https://ebookcentral.proquest.com

Sue, D. W., & Torino, G. C. (2005). Racial-cultural competence: Awareness, knowledge, and skills. In R. T. Carter (Ed.), *Handbook of racial-cultural psychology and counseling:* Vol. 2. *Training and practice* (pp. 3–18). Hoboken, NJ: John Wiley & Sons Inc.

Sutcliffe, K. M., Lewton, E., & Rosenthal, M. M. (2004). Communication failures: An insidious contributor to medical mishaps. *Academic Medicine, 79*(2), 186–194. https://doi.org/10.1097/00001888-200402000-00019

Taylor, R. (2008). *The intentional relationship: Occupational therapy and use of self.* Philadelphia, PA: FA Davis.

Trzeciak, S., Mazzarelli, A., & Booker, C. (2019). *Compassionomics: The revolutionary scientific evidence that caring makes a difference.* Pensacola, FL: Studer Group.

Ulrey, K. L., & Amason, P. (2001). Intercultural communication between patients and health care providers: An exploration of intercultural communication effectiveness, cultural sensitivity, stress, and anxiety. *Health Communication, 13*(4), 449–463. https://doi.org/10.1207/s15327027hc1304_06

U.S. Department of Health and Human Services (USDHSS) (2003). *Developing cultural competence in disaster mental health programs: Guiding principles and recommendations* (DHHS Pub. No. SMA 3828). Rockville, MD: Center for Mental Health Services. Substance Abuse and Mental Health Services Administration. https://store.samhsa.gov/sites/default/files/d7/priv/sma11-disaster-01.pdf

Wampold, B. E., & Brown, G. S. J. (2005). Estimating variability in outcomes attributable to therapists: A naturalistic study of outcomes in managed care. *Journal of Consulting and Clinical Psychology, 73*(5), 914. https://doi.org/10.1037/0022-006x.73.5.914

Wells, S. A., Black, R. B., & Gupta, J. (2016). *Culture and occupation: Effectiveness for occupational therapy practice, education, and research* (3rd ed.). Bethesda, MD: AOTA Press.

Woolf, S. H., Kuzel, A. J., Dovey, S. M., & Phillips, R. L. (2004). A string of mistakes: The importance of cascade analysis in describing, counting, and preventing medical errors. *The Annals of Family Medicine, 2*(4), 317–326. https://doi.org/10.1370/afm.126

2

A MODEL FOR TRANSFORMING RACIAL AND CULTURAL LINES

Listening, loving, and lifting spirits

Complexities of listening

VIGNETTE 2.1 TRANSFORMING RACIAL AND CULTURAL LINES

Martha, a 75-year-old African American female, had recently lost her beloved husband of 50 years to the coronavirus and was forced to live in a residential care centre. The facility's RN, Samuel, asked how she was adjusting. Martha expressed how much she missed her partner and how she felt deeply isolated living in an all-white residential facility. "I am not only broken-hearted about my husband, but I am so damn lonely here. It is like I am invisible – no one sees me except the few Black CNAs and janitors. To everyone else, I do not exist. When I do share what is in my heart, the CNAs and janitors look like they are listening. The white residents appear to be distracted or doing something else. They listen to me with their ears and not their heart. I want them to listen to know me – just like you are right now."

Although every aspect of communication has the potential to support human connection, exploring the complexity of listening provides a unique portal towards developing the multiple dimensions of flexible, caring, and effective communication. As Joseph Alpert, a medical professor and cardiologist noted, "the most common failure in communicating information is the result of inattentive or inaccurate listening" (Alpert, 2011, p. 381). Patients have ranked "listening" as the most important behaviour of health professionals (Harris & Templeton, 2001). As is evident in Martha's story in vignette 2.1, listening well and showing how much we care, is at the heart of client-centred care. It is only when we offer our aware presence and skilful engaged listening that we can be open to the depth of our client's true concerns and can begin forging a partnership towards healing. In order to provide optimal care, it is equally important for diverse members of health and social care teams to communicate well with each other (Kleiner et al., 2014; Leonard et al., 2004; Sargeant et al., 2008; Sargeant et al., 2011).

On one level, listening is a very simple and basic skill. A person simply decides to be present to genuinely hear what another person has to say by keeping their own mind free of distractions, choosing not to interrupt the other person with their own stories or advice, and allowing for silence. On another level, listening is very profound and complex. It can be challenging to keep one's mind free of distractions, especially if one has not been listened to in a while. It can be hard not to interrupt someone speaking, especially when there are time and performance pressures, when emotions are triggered, or when a story reminds us of our own experience. It can be difficult to allow for a silence that informs, especially if this was never modelled in our own family, our racial or cultural group, or from our professional training. We can be challenged to maintain our focus when our clients', patients', or team members' stories are painful or emotional; especially when we have had a busy, demanding workday and simply have run out of attention. It can be hard to listen because racial and cultural differences may feel unfamiliar or uncomfortable.

When clients are invited to share their concerns, they may be hesitant to disclose much or reveal deeply about themselves because we are putting our attention on taking notes instead of what is being shared. Our facial expressions may show too much worry, too much fear, or too much concern for someone to open up about a traumatic event. Instead, they may need a relaxed, confident, and caring expression on our face or some quick-witted humour that expresses our common humanity. The experience of too much eye contact may be a problem for someone from a racial or cultural group that reserves the intimacy of eye contact only for very familiar people. Our posture may not be inviting to the person speaking, and if we are fidgeting – this could be distracting to someone attempting to identify and share areas where they need assistance. Racial, cultural, and socio-economic class differences may contribute to a patient or member of the health care team not trusting that someone from a different background can actually hear, identify, and be present with their concerns. These are just a few of the intricacies that can affect communication exchanges and in particular, impact the effectiveness of our listening.

Educational interventions to improve communication skills for health and social care practitioners

Given that the communication skills of practitioners are not innate and do not necessarily improve over time or with clinical experience (Fallowfield et al., 2002; Moore et al., 2018), many educational interventions and courses now train health professionals to be more effective and compassionate communicators. *Oncotalk*, developed by medical faculty at Duke University, the University of Pittsburgh, and other medical schools, teaches oncology fellows clinical empathy and listening skills in a 5-day intensive retreat (Back et al., 2007; Boodman, 2015). Columbia University developed a programme in narrative medicine that emphasizes the importance of listening and understanding a patient's life story (Charon, 2001). Twenty years ago, Dr Remen and her colleagues created a course for first- and second-year medical students at the University of California San Francisco called "The Healer's Art". This course, now in 70 of the medical schools in the United States, emphasizes that the best practice of medicine and health services is about connecting with patients and clients, a process which requires more listening than doing, and focuses on evoking the inner strength within patients and clients to respond to their health challenges (Rabow et al., 2007; Remen Institute for the Study of Health and Illness, n.d.). Faculty at the University of Illinois in Chicago train medical students to ask questions and listen for important contextual information related to race, religion, socioeconomic class, and other cultural variables that impact health in standardized patients (Schwartz et al., 2010; Weiner & Schwartz, 2015).

While lectures have limited value in teaching and in practising communication skills, key active learning strategies that yield improvements include the use of standardized patients or Objective Structured Clinical Examination (OSCE), role-play, videotapes, skill practice, feedback, multidisciplinary panels, reflective journals, small group discussion, and interactive theatre (Banerjee et al., 2017; Berkhof et al., 2011; Boschma et al., 2010; Nikmanesh et al., 2018; O'Sullivan et al., 2008; Sargeant et al., 2011; Shield et al., 2011). While praised for their effectiveness, educational interventions that require standardized patients and intensive retreats have also been criticized for being time- and resource-intensive.

The use of Google Chat, a free online instant messaging program, has been piloted to support the use of role-playing, reflection, and feedback that contribute to the enhancement of communication skills fostered between pairs of physicians. After basics on communication skills are reviewed, participants are asked to complete an online role-play session (one as a patient or family member, another as a physician) with a facilitator observing the conversation online and providing feedback. Participants favourably reviewed Google Chat for its convenience and sustainability as a method for improving their communication skills (Saraiya & Avvento, 2013). Zoom, GoToMeeting, Skype Meet Now, Jitsi Meet, GlobalMeet Collaboration, and many others are increasingly used as educational tools for enhancing the communication skills of health and social care practitioners.

Listening partnerships: An innovative, sustainable, educational intervention for developing effective communication

Froehlich and colleagues at the University of New England have explored the use of a particular tool, *listening partnerships*, for developing strong listening skills as the foundation for culturally and racially effective communication (Froehlich, 2017; Froehlich & Nesbit, 2004; Froehlich et al., 2014; Froehlich et al., 2016). Listening partnerships are based on the theory and practice of re-evaluation counselling, also known as co-counselling (Jackins, 1981; Kauffman & New, 2004). In listening partnerships, pairs or small groups of peers agree to exchange confidential listening, generally for an equal amount of time each. Potential topics suggested for discussion include the ups and downs of everyday life, life stories, goals, stressors, leisure interests, experiences as health and social care students and practitioners, and experiences related to race, gender, class, culture, disability, and other constituencies.

Although the use of standardized patients and role-play is effective in teaching communication skills to practitioners, there is no substitute for authentic human interaction in the development of listening, empathy, and compassion. Some practitioners report that it can feel stiff and scripted to show compassion and caring towards a trained actor. Although listening partnerships in dyads and groups may feel stiff initially, with practice, listening partnerships offer an opportunity to develop communication skills in a non-scripted and authentic setting. In addition, costs are minimal, and partners can meet at a time that is convenient for them. Listening partnerships offer a confidential opportunity to strengthen connections with peers and improve communication through the provision of supportive feedback. Hence, this book will emphasize the process of exchanging engaged listening with peers, in pairs or small groups, as a readily available, sustainable, and effective method of developing multiple facets of one's communication skills, and at the same time, developing a peer support network. While learning to listen with our full attention is at the heart of successful listening partnerships, it is critical to explore additional nuances of effective communication by beginning with a self-assessment of one's strengths and areas for improvement when communicating with racially and culturally diverse people (see Appendix B, "Assessing your strengths and areas for improvement as a racially and culturally effective communicator" for several surveys).

Froehlich Communication Survey

The Froehlich Communication Survey (see Appendix B, Table 1) is noted by practitioners and students for raising awareness of the communication skills they already possess and the skills they would like to improve. It has good test-retest reliability and internal consistency (Cronbach's alpha =.847). An interprofessional panel of experts from nursing, social work, counselling, occupational therapy, and osteopathic medicine contributed to the refinement and content validity of the instrument. It has been shown to be a useful tool in evaluating health professional students' perceptions of their communication skills before and after exposure to an interprofessional communication curriculum (Froehlich et al., 2016). A brief version of this survey is also included in Appendix B (see Appendix B, Table 2).

Treasuring the Human Race Survey

Thornton-Marsh and Froehlich developed the Treasuring the Human Race Survey (see Appendix B, Table 3) to engage the reader in the transformational, creative, and liberating process of noticing their complete goodness as a human and in identifying goals related to racial-cultural awareness, competence, and humility. Readers reflect on their awareness and appreciation of different racial groups so they can identify action steps to take on the journey towards embracing racial diversity and transforming racial lines. Components of this survey are also embedded in the Racial and Cultural Awareness and Action Survey.

Racial and Cultural Awareness and Action Survey

The Racial and Cultural Awareness and Action Survey (see Appendix B, Table 4) prompts the reader to assess their understanding of the historical context, strengths, and challenges of many racial and cultural groups and to identify action steps they can take to be more culturally effective. Although psychometric properties have not yet been established, the survey content has been validated by social workers, occupational therapists, educators, and counsellors from diverse backgrounds. Health practitioners and students state that they value the survey because it increases their awareness of the racial and cultural groups they need to learn more about, and helps them identify steps to take in order to be racially and culturally effective practitioners.

Treasuring All Life Survey

Given the global threat of climate change to the health and wellbeing of all humans, but particularly to People of the Global Majority (PGM) and communities of colour, the Treasuring All Life Survey (see Appendix B, Table 5) invites the reader to explore the moral imperative of joining together within and across racial and cultural lines to honour, preserve, sustain, and restore all life on the planet. Similar to engaging with the Treasuring the Human Race Survey, engaging with the Treasuring All Life Survey is a transformational, creative, and liberating process. The purpose of this survey is to help you notice your complete goodness, intelligence, and power as a human and to identify goals related to treasuring all life so you can join across racial and cultural lines to take action towards the flourishing of all life.

Evaluation of listening partnerships

Froehlich and colleagues have used listening partnerships in a graduate occupational therapy programme for a number of years with positive reviews by students from diverse backgrounds (Froehlich, 2010, 2017; Froehlich & Nesbit, 2004; Froehlich et al., 2016). See Table 2.1 for student and practitioner comments about listening partnerships.

TABLE 2.1 Reflections on listening partnerships

Student comments

"Listening partnerships were helpful in that feedback was given in a constructive manner. It gave me a safe place to practice my communication skills and to discuss what I could do better."

"At the beginning of listening partnerships, I was really nervous and became closed off when talking about certain subjects. As I have become more familiar with my listening partner and staying committed to bettering my communication, I feel more comfortable expressing my ideas. Also, I have become a stronger listener through increased competence by asking open-ended questions and allowing for silences due to having multiple conversations with my listening partner."

"I was already a good listener, but listening partnerships helped me talk because I am quiet. They gave me the confidence to talk. They also helped me build friendships with other students of color and white students."

"As a woman of color, there were many times that I needed to step out of my comfort zone to converse with students I did not know too well. At first, I did not like it, but eventually, I embraced it because I believe that it actually made me a better communicator (speaker and listener). Eventually, I was able to listen for meaning and decipher the most important content of the conversation. We discovered commonalities between us – past experiences, stresses with school, and family values … this fostered trust in our relationships."

Practitioner comments

"Practicing the art of listening through listening partnerships truly taught me how to be in the moment. Too often I would catch my mind wandering during daily conversations with friends and family rather than be fully devoted to the exchange at hand. These assignments not only showed me the importance of truly hearing and listening to a person; they allowed me to refine my effective communication skills for my personal life and clinical practice."

Froehlich, 2017, p. 86

"These partnerships have taught me multiple tools that I carry with me to this day and know that I will carry and take with me throughout my professional career. Being able to listen to my clients as well as co-workers makes for a better, safer, and more effective environment."

Froehlich, 2017, p. 86

Using a pre-test, post-test design, Froehlich and colleagues (2016) evaluated the influence of listening partnerships on undergraduate student ratings of their own communication skills in an interprofessional introduction to health professions course. In both the intervention and control groups, students were exposed to an established communication curriculum that included interactive learning activities related to cultural competence and listening skills; teamwork and assertiveness; obtaining a health history; and motivational interviewing. While both groups were introduced to listening partnerships, the intervention group engaged in weekly practice with 2–3 minutes of listening partnerships. Both groups showed a significant improvement in self-perceptions of their verbal and non-verbal communication as measured by mean scores out of 100 on Froehlich's survey ($p<.001$). While 16 out of 25 items on the survey were significantly influenced by both curricula, only the intervention group showed a significant difference in their perceived ability to listen with compassion ($p<.05$). Given the debate in health care literature about whether or not compassion can be taught, this is an important finding. Perhaps participation in the exchange of engaged listening among members of health and social care teams, in contrast to all the one-way attention practitioners provide to their patients and clients, can diminish the tremendous compassion fatigue noted in health care.

A model for transforming racial and cultural lines: Listening, loving, and lifting spirits

Given the value of deepening awareness of racial and cultural lines while engaging in listening partnerships in dyads and groups to build the capacity to listen and connect within and across racial and cultural lines, the authors propose a model for transforming these lines to optimize the delivery of health and social care with confidential, engaged listening at the centre of this work (see Figure 2.1). Taking turns

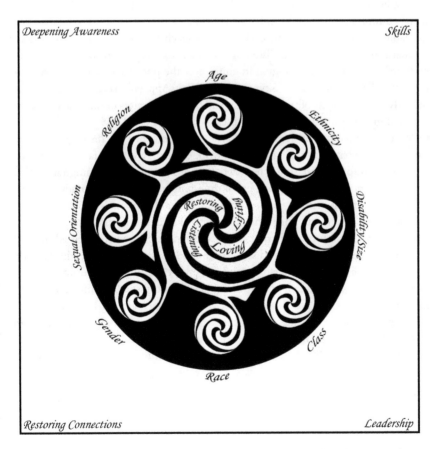

FIGURE 2.1 A model for transforming racial and cultural lines in health and social care

listening with caring and compassion is the distinct feature of listening partnerships. This process enables practitioners and students to increase their awareness and sense of aliveness in themselves and others and to build the skills of listening, loving, and lifting spirits with diverse groups of people. Partnerships that transcend the countless divisions that exist in society will generate creative action towards achieving optimal health and wellbeing for humans. Leadership that fosters unity within and across racial and cultural lines generates the vital life force that holds promise in addressing the interrelationship between the health of the planet, the health of humankind, and the flourishing of all life.

Establishing listening partnerships

Once readers have completed the Froehlich Communication Survey, the Treasuring the Human Race Survey, the Racial and Cultural Awareness and Action Survey, and the Treasuring All Life Survey, it is recommended that they share their results (strengths, areas for improvement, and goals) with a listening partner or partners. Ideally, listening partners are individuals who are also reading this book to improve their communication skills and can commit to engaging in several listening exchanges, ideally a minimum of 10 minutes each way with additional time for feedback and discussion after listening has been exchanged. Although in-person partnerships are ideal, exchanging listening over the phone or through video conferencing (FaceTime, Zoom, Skype, Signal, WhatsApp, etc.) is also effective – particularly in the context of transportation and distance barriers or physical distancing required in the context of infectious diseases such as COVID-19.

Whether meeting in person or via teleconference technology, listening partnerships in triads or small groups can work extremely well. In fact, some people are more comfortable sharing when two or more people are listening rather than one. The principle of exchanging equal time remains the same in triads and small groups. Identifying primary and secondary listeners helps triads and small groups function well. When only the primary listener asks questions and shares comments, the person taking a turn at sharing their experiences can remain focused in triads or small groups. The secondary listeners' undivided attention and feedback at the conclusion of listening partnerships tend to be very useful and appreciated.

Establishing confidentiality is one of the keys to successful listening partnerships. Listening partners are asked not to disclose anything partners have shared in a listening partnership outside the partnership. In addition, listening partners are asked not to bring up anything previously shared in a listening partnership with a listening partner without first checking in to see whether his or her partner would like to revisit a particular topic raised. These two types of confidentiality create the conditions for listening partners to open up to each other both about what is going well in their lives and to share the challenges they are facing. While there are benefits to exchanging listening with a variety of listening partners, readers are encouraged over time to identify individuals who can be regular listening partners.

Engaging in listening partnerships both within and across racial and cultural lines will accelerate the development of culturally effective communication.

At the conclusion of a listening partnership session, it is generally useful for the listener to ask their partner questions to get their attention off their session and onto the present-time reality that life is good. This skill will be addressed in Chapter 6 ("Lifting spirits") in the section on attention off distress, redirection, and celebrating the present. In this way, the person who was listened to will now be ready to be the listener. As was noted, it will also be important at the conclusion of many listening partnerships to exchange feedback on what the listener did well and what could have made the session go even better. The sensitive nature of giving and receiving feedback will be revisited in Chapter 7 ("Teamwork and collaboration").

A walk through listening partnerships

Once two or more individuals have made an agreement to engage in listening partnerships to improve their communication skills, they will find it helpful to have a number of discussion topics (see Tables 1–6 in Appendix C: "Listening and engaging to transform: Listening partnership questions and discussion/journal prompts"). Table C.1 ("Partnerships on the art of effective communication within and across racial and cultural lines") provides a variety of potential topics not only for listening partnerships, but also for journalling and discussion that are aimed at assisting learners in connecting with each other as they develop and reflect upon communication skills identified in the Froehlich Communication Survey. Additional tables (Table C.2, "Partnerships to support understanding racial and cultural identities and experiences with oppression"; Table C.3, "Partnerships to build alliances and pride within and across racial and cultural lines"; Table C.4, "Partnerships for deeper and restorative connections and understanding"; Table C.5, "Partnerships to support listening in health and social care teams: Voices of frontline workers as leaders"; and Table C.6, "Partnerships to embolden leadership") provide potential topics for listening partnerships, discussion, and journalling that are relevant for further developing racially and culturally responsive communication. Listening partnership questions and discussion/journal prompts for dialogue, reflection, connection, and transformation are also embedded in each chapter.

References

Alpert, J. (2011). Some simple rules for effective communication in clinical teaching and practice environments. *The American Journal of Medicine, 124*(5), 381–382. www.amjmed.com/article/S0002-9343(11)00058-1/fulltext

Back, A. L., Arnold, R. M., Baile, W. F., Fryer-Edwards, K. A., Alexander, S. C., Barley, G. E., … Tulsky, J. A. (2007). Efficacy of communication skills training for giving bad news and discussing transitions to palliative care. *Archives of Internal Medicine, 167*(5), 453–460. https://doi.org/10.1001/archinte.167.5.453

Banerjee, S. C., Manna, R., Coyle, N., Penn, S., Gallegos, T. E., Zaider, T., … Parker, P. A. (2017). The implementation and evaluation of a communication skills training program for oncology nurses. *Translational Behavioral Medicine, 7*(3), 615–623. https://doi.org/10.1007/s13142-017-0473-5

Berkhof, M., van Rijssen, J., Schellart, A. J., Anema, J. R., & van der Beek, A. J. (2011). Effective training strategies for teaching communication skills to physicians: An overview of systematic reviews. *Patient Education Counseling, 84*(2) 152–162. https://doi.org/10.1016/j.pec.2010.06.010

Boodman, S. (2015, March 9). Teaching doctors how to engage more and lecture less. *The Washington Post.* www.washingtonpost.com/national/health-science/teaching-doctors-how-to-engage-more-and-lecture-less/2015/03/09/95a98508-ae30-11e4-9c91-e9d2f9fde644_story.html

Boschma, G., Einboden, R., Groening, M., Jackson, C., MacPhee, M., Marshall, H., … Roberts, E. (2010). Strengthening communication education in an undergraduate nursing curriculum. *International Journal of Nursing Education Scholarship, 7*(1), 1–14. https://doi.org/10.2202/1548-923x.2043

Charon, R. (2001). Narrative medicine: A model for empathy, reflection, profession, and trust. *Journal of the American Medical Association, 286*(15), 1897–1902. https://doi.org/10.1001/jama.286.15.1897

Fallowfield, L., Jenkins, V., Farewell, V., Saul, J., Duffy, A., & Eves, R. (2002). Efficacy of a Cancer Research UK communication skills training model for oncologists: A randomized controlled trial. *The Lancet, 359*(9307), 650–656. https://doi.org/10.1016/s0140-6736(02)07810-8

Froehlich, J. (2010). Effective communication. In K. Sladyk, K. Jacobs, & N. MacRae (Eds), *Occupational therapy essentials for clinical competence* (pp. 331–344). Thorofare, NJ: SLACK, Inc.

Froehlich, J. (2017). Effective communication. In K. Jacobs & N. MacRae (Eds), *Occupational therapy essentials for clinical competence* (3rd ed., pp. 99–132). Thorofare, NJ: SLACK, Inc.

Froehlich, J., & Nesbit, S. (2004). The aware communicator: Dialogues on diversity. *Occupational Therapy in Health Care, 18*(1–2), 171–182. https://doi.org/10.1080/J003v18n01_16

Froehlich, J., Pardue, K., & Dunbar, D. S. (2016). Evaluation of a communication survey and interprofessional education curriculum for undergraduate health professional students. *Health and Interprofessional Practice, 2*(4), eP1082. https://hipe-pub.org/articles/abstract/10.7772/2159-1253.1082/

Froehlich, J., Roy, M. C., Augustoni, B., Arsenault, A., & Eldredge, J. (2014). Effective communication. In K. Jacobs & N. MacRae (Eds), *Occupational therapy essentials for clinical competence* (2nd ed., pp. 85–112). Thorofare, NJ: SLACK, Inc.

Harris, S. R., & Templeton, E. (2001). Who's listening? Experiences of women with breast cancer in communicating with physicians. *The Breast Journal, 7*(6), 444–469. https://doi.org/10.1046/j.1524-4741.2001.07614.x

Jackins, H. (1981). *The art of listening.* Seattle, WA: Rational Island Publishers.

Kauffman, K., & New, C. (2004). *Co-counseling: The theory and practice of re-evaluation counseling.* Hove, UK: Brunner-Routledge.

Kleiner, C., Link, T., Travis Maynard, M., & Carpenter, K. H. (2014). Coaching to improve the quality of communication during briefings and debriefings. *Association of periOperative Registered Nurses Journal, 100*(4), 358–368. doi: 10.1016/j.aorn.2014.03.012

Leonard, M., Graham, S., & Bonacum, D. (2004). The human factor: The critical import-ance of effective teamwork and communication in providing safe care. *Quality Safe Care, 13*(Suppl. 1), i85–i90. https://doi.org/10.1136/qshc.2004.010033

Moore, P. M., Rivera, S., Bravo-Soto, G. A., Olivares, C., & Lawrie, T. A. (2018). Communication skills training for healthcare professionals working with people who have cancer. Cochrane Database of Systematic Reviews, 7, article CD003751. Doi: 10.1002/14651858.CD003751.pub4

Nikmanesh, P., Mohammadzadeh, B., Nobakht, S., & Yusefi, A. R. (2018). Nurses commu-nication skills training and its effect on patients' satisfaction in teaching hospitals of Shiraz University of Medical Sciences. *Iranian Journal of Health Science, 6*(4), 22–29. https://doi.org/10.18502/jhs.v6i4.201

O'Sullivan, P., Chao, S., Russell, M., Levine, S., & Fabiny, A. (2008). Development and imple-mentation of an objective structured clinical examination to provide formative feedback on communication and interpersonal skills in geriatric training. *Journal of the American Geriatric Society, 56*, 1730–1735. https://doi.org/10.1111/j.1532-5415.2008.01860.x

Rabow, M. W., Wrubel, J., & Remen, R. N. (2007). Authentic community as an educa-tional strategy for advancing professionalism: A national evaluation of The Healer's Art course. *Journal of General Internal Medicine, 22*(10), 1422–1428. https://doi.org/10.1007/s11606-007-0274-5

Remen Institute for the Study of Health and Illness (RISHI). (n.d.). Healer's Art overview. www.rishiprograms.org/healers-art/

Saraiya, B., & Avvento, P. (2013). Google Chat as an online innovative, personalized com-munication skills training program. *Journal of Pain and Symptom Management, 45*(2), 389.

Sargeant, J., Loney, E., & Murphy, G. (2008). Effective interprofessional teams: "Contact is not enough" to build a team. *Journal of Continuing Education in the Health Professions, 28*(4), 228–234. https://doi.org/10.1002/chp.189

Sargeant, J., MacLeod, T., & Murray, A. (2011). An interprofessional approach to teaching communication skills. *Journal of Continuing Education in the Health Professions, 31*(4) 265–267. https://doi.org/10.1002/chp.20139

Schwartz, A., Weiner, S. J., Harris, I. B., & Binns-Calvey, A. (2010). An educational inter-vention for contextualizing patient care and medical students' abilities to probe for con-textual issues in simulated patients. *Journal of the American Medical Association, 304*(11), 1191–1197. https://doi.org/10.1001/jama.2010.1297

Shield, R. R., Tong, I., Tomas, M., & Besdine, R. W. (2011). Teaching communication and compassionate care skills: An innovative curriculum for pre-clerkship medical students. *Medical Teacher, 33*, e408–e416. https://doi.org/10.3109/0142159x.2011.586748

Weiner, S., & Schwartz, A. (2015). *Listening for what matters: Avoiding contextual errors in health care.* London: Oxford University Press.

PART II

Refinement of racially and culturally effective communication in health and social care

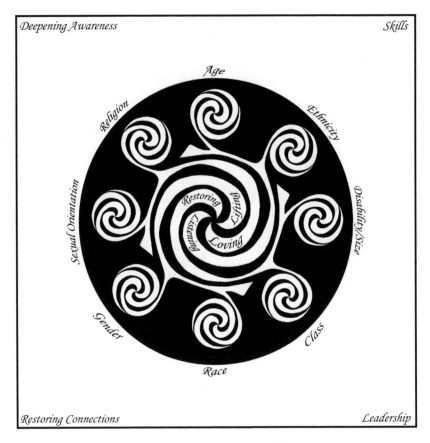

FIGURE 3.1 A model for transforming racial and cultural lines in health and social care

PART II MODEL COMPONENTS SKILLS: LISTENING, LOVING, AND LIFTING SPIRITS

- Presence and attunement
- Loving and inviting life narratives
- Aligning and responding to thoughts and emotions
- Lifting spirits
- Teamwork and collaboration

3

PRESENCE AND ATTUNEMENT

Not interrupting

VIGNETTE 3.1 HONOURING THE FLOW: 流れを尊重する NAGARE O SONCHŌ SURU

Satchiko, a middle-aged Japanese woman, presented with a long list of symptoms that had been compiled over anxiety-filled days and terror-filled nights. The physical therapist, Phyllis, was practised at being able to keep up with the pacing of Satchiko's expression of the concerns she had been experiencing with her arthritis. Satchiko talked quickly, punctuating parts of her description with examples of her fears, highlights, and worries. Phyllis called this kind of listening to Satchiko "honouring the flow" which discouraged any questions being asked while Satchiko shared, and encouraged a receptivity and welcoming of all that needed to be shared.

VIGNETTE 3.2 REFRAINING FROM OFFERING ADVICE

While working on an inpatient psychiatric unit, Julie was able to learn first-hand what it was like to have a conversation without even speaking. Julie was working with Mark, a white working-class man, who was suffering from drug addiction. Julie introduced herself and explained her role as Mark's occupational therapist and her role in his plan of care, but before Julie could explain any further, Mark began describing his dilemmas and family problems and before the session was over, Mark had solved his problems without advice. "Well, I guess all I needed to do

> *was just think it all through," said Mark. Even though Julie did not offer professional advice or problem solving, Mark was able to think through his thoughts and actions without being interrupted and took charge of his own problem-solving strategies.*
>
> *Froehlich, 2017, p. 105*

As Jackins (1981) noted, frequent interruptions characterize much of human interactions. Beckman and Frankel's (1984) iconic study found that physicians in the United States interrupted patients after a mere 18 seconds of patients beginning to explain their problems. Follow-up studies found that physicians listened for 23 seconds before interrupting (Marvel et al., 1999) and residents interrupted an average of 12 seconds after entering the room of a patient (Rhoades et al., 2001). Danczak (2015) found that in Britain, where doctors receive specific training in how to listen without interrupting at the start of a consultation, general practitioners hardly interrupted at all and generally allowed patients to complete their opening statements, which usually took less than a minute. The average time before an interruption occurred was 47 seconds and 88% of patients were able to express their main concern within 5 minutes.

Whether the health or social care practitioner is conducting an initial interview, assessment, intake, or engaging in ongoing exchanges with their clients, there is a time and place for interruptions for promoting an interactional process of "give and take". However, given the human tendency to interrupt each other, there is a valuable place for learning to "bite one's tongue" and to be fully present as we allow another person to finish his or her process of sharing thoughts and emotions. As Danczak (2015) noted, interrupting patients or clients may mean that important issues do not emerge, and practitioners run the risk of errors in assuming they already know a patient's concerns if they are in a hurry to stop listening and start talking. Additionally, studies have shown that listening to patients at the start of a consultation does not lead to longer consultations (Joos et al., 1996; Putnam et al., 1988). The significance of listening without interruption for the provision of optimal care is highlighted by Phyllis and Julie in vignettes 3.1 and 3.2.

Keeping one's mind free of distractions and silence

VIGNETTE 3.3 INNER QUIET: الهدوء الداخل ALHUDU' ALDDAKHILIU

Silence is the space that opens up between a practitioner and patient where stillness can be honoured and the noise from the pressure of a busy outpatient clinic can be muted and released. Wahidah, NP, relished the moments where she allowed the inner quiet within her to prevail and not the urgent external pressure to see the next patient. She encouraged its presence in the space between herself and Muhammad, a Lebanese patient who felt respected by her silence; a silence that honoured being with him and which enabled him to trust her. There is nothing more significant than being versus doing.

VIGNETTE 3.4 SILENCE: σιωπή SIOPÍ

Ali, an occupational therapist, was working in an outpatient paediatric clinic and had been treating a young Greek boy, Lucas, for gravitational insecurity. They had been working together for a few weeks when she had the opportunity to consult with both his mother and father after a treatment session. She simply asked, "How are things going?" At first, their responses were broad, but as Ali allowed for silence, Lucas's parents began to express new concerns they had not yet shared with her. She learned that Lucas had only slept in his own bed a handful of times throughout his life – which was tiresome and frustrating for both him and his parents. Ali collaborated with the family to incorporate this new information into a revised plan of care.

Froehlich, 2017, p. 105

By allowing for silence and providing their full attention to their clients, Wahidah and Ali, in vignettes 3.3 and 3.4, built rapport and learned key information. For centuries, Indigenous people have used talking circles for important gatherings in which each participant is listened to without interruption, and silence is welcomed – sometimes a talking stick is used to hold the sacred space for only one person to share information and be honoured at a time. Though non-indigenous people should not appropriate Indigenous culture by incorporating talking sticks into a listening process, the use of other objects and a timer can be helpful in dividing listening time and speaking time. One can practise not interrupting and instead become fully present, engaged, mindful, and aware as a listener. Knowing that you, as a listener, will also have a chance to be heard by your listening partner can curtail interruptions because there is a space for your thoughts as well.

Given that the human mind has a tendency to wander, keeping one's mind free of distractions and being fully present while listening can be challenging. Mindfulness has been described as paying attention on purpose in the present moment with kindness and without judgment (Kabat-Zinn, 2009). Training in mindfulness, loving thoughtfulness, and/or conscious presence can be facilitated through meditation, breathing, and yoga. These practices promote the process of mindful listening. When we notice our minds wandering as we are listening, it is important to bring our minds back, without judgment, to what is being shared by the person who is speaking (Shafir, 2003). This process can be greatly enhanced when we are also listened to by others who are also reaching to be fully present, mindful listeners. When both people take turns holding the space for each other, a truly honouring process evolves.

Exchanging one minute each way of listening

After discussing the survey results (Froehlich Communication Survey, Treasuring the Human Race Survey, Racial and Cultural Awareness and Action Survey, and Treasuring All Life Survey) with a listening partner or partners, it will be useful to have a first listening partnership that is brief – 1 minute each way to practise not interrupting and mindful listening. In this, and *only* in this partnership, the listener is asked to say nothing. Topics for the first listening partnership can include why you want to be a health or social care practitioner or what communication patterns were like in your family. These topics and many others listed in Appendix C can facilitate listening in this first partnership.

After exchanging 1 minute of listening, it is important to discuss what it was like to be a listener who did not speak and to be the speaker who was just listened to.

- Was it difficult to be quiet and say nothing as a listener? If so, was it useful to practise stopping and thinking before saying anything in the role of the listener?
- As a listener, were you able to give your full attention and presence to your partner or was your mind busy with thoughts such as how you were doing as a listener, how you felt about the person you listened to, how awkward this type of exchange was, or any other concerns?
- What was the experience like to speak for 1 minute while your partner just listened?
- Did you enjoy the opportunity to have someone "just listen", or did you need verbal encouragement to continue talking?
- Did racial or cultural factors influence your experience of listening without distractions and of sharing and being listened to without interruptions?

In a 1-minute listening partnership, you may not have the opportunities to face many distracting thoughts as a listener or the experiences to allow for silences. However, there will be plenty of opportunities in future listening partnerships to practise the art of allowing for silences and keeping one's mind free of distractions. Although it is sometimes a bit awkward to allow for silences, just the right amount of quiet space can allow a person speaking to gather his or her thoughts and feelings and continue sharing. The speaker may discover important insights when a listener can offer a silent, relaxed, caring space. On the other hand, too much silence may indicate that the speaker needs encouragement, validation, or a thoughtful question from the person listening to continue sharing.

Attunement: The significance of non-verbal communication

VIGNETTE 3.5 WITHOUT WORDS: SENZA PAROLE

Marie, an occupational therapist, was working with a client with dementia who was a fluent speaker of English, but began to speak her first language, Italian. Although Marie did not understand Italian, the more she offered her eye contact and warm facial expression, the more animated her client became. The family reported they hadn't seen that level of animation in a long time. Eventually, she grabbed Marie's arm and was ready to walk again. She hadn't walked without her walker in many weeks. Marie attributes her client's progress to her skilled non-verbal communication.

Froehlich, 2017, pp. 107–109

VIGNETTE 3.6 ATTUNEMENT: SINTONIZACIÓN

Juanito, a middle-aged Puerto Rican man, expressed the loneliness of being in a marriage where he felt unheard, ignored, and unloved. During their first counselling session, Timaya, MSW, encouraged Juanito and his wife, Carmela, to initiate and maintain loving eye contact, without speaking words. Juanito began to cry deeply and shared that he felt Carmela was finally seeing him. Carmela conveyed that she was present, that she was interested, and that she valued Juanito. Her loving gaze began to dissolve the barriers that had separated them from each other. Through their eyes, they searched for each other in a moment of human connection. Unbeknownst to Juanito and Carmela, Timaya was also gazing lovingly at both of them as she silently was moved by their connection and presence with one another.

Practitioner vignettes 3.5 and 3.6 highlight the powerful role non-verbal communication can play in being attuned and aligned with others. Attunement is a process achieved by being aware of our connection to each other and by being attentive to every profound moment where we non-verbally reach out to one another and communicate on a level deeper than words. It is a process where we allow for and are open to communicating and to connecting on the levels of noticing, sensing, interpreting, and understanding from the heart. Attunement is intuitive in that it is more than the five senses. It is the human exchange of energy we are born with. This process is fluid, in the moment, reciprocal, possibly subconscious, aware or unaware, intentional, or unintentional. When we are not attuned and are blocked from this source of connection, non-verbal communication can be misunderstood, awkward, and off-putting – particularly across racial and cultural lines.

Offering our non-verbal expression

The warmth of our smile, kindness in our eyes, an inviting tone of voice, and attentive posture can often convey more than any words or verbal expressions we share as practitioners. Yet a flexible, creative, and attuned listener explores a multitude of variations in eye contact, tone of voice, and posture to evoke a mutuality of connection with any given client.

As a general guideline, it is important for a listener to have his or her gaze available for someone they are listening to. Individuals sharing important concerns may or may not feel comfortable making eye contact while they speak, but most people will derive reassurance from knowing that the listener's eye contact is available. On the other hand, there will be situations where sitting side by side will allow a client to feel more comfortable and able to share.

Early in the practice of listening partnerships, it may be difficult for listeners not to fidget. Froehlich et al. (2016) found that refraining from fidgeting had the lowest initial scores for undergraduate health professions students as indicated in the Froehlich Communication Survey. Nonetheless, students in both an established and experimental curriculum showed significantly higher scores on this item in post-surveys after exposure to an intentional curriculum with active learning strategies and some exposure to listening partnerships. This parallels Froehlich's findings in teaching graduate occupational therapy students. Often with just one reminder, students learn to discontinue tapping a pen, shaking their leg, nodding too frequently, handling a coffee cup, or twirling their hair while they are in the listener role. Many were completely unaware of their fidgeting behaviour. Some students report they are just too jittery to sit still when they are initially learning to listen and find they can tap a toe to quietly release tension in a way that is not obvious or distracting to the listener. With repeated practice in listening partnerships, the need to fidget at all tends to disappear.

Receiving non-verbal expressions

Besides being aware and creative in communicating non-verbally, being attuned to the nuances of non-verbal communication in others deepens and clarifies our understanding of emotions and the deeper meaning underlying what is being shared verbally. For example, what does posture tell us? Is our client standing or sitting proudly or are they slumped and showing discouragement or hopelessness? Is their tone of voice confident or does it betray anxiety or defensiveness? Is there a quiver of the lips or a smiling relaxed facial expression? Do the words our clients share match their non-verbal communication? Is there a ring in someone's voice when they address a particular experience or concern? The aware and attuned communicator notes multiple dimensions of both verbal and non-verbal communication to discern what is most important to the speaker and responds flexibly to what is shared.

To mirror or not to mirror non-verbal communication

VIGNETTE 3.7 INVISIBLE ENERGY

Ruth, a white woman living in poverty, was mandated by the courts to attend case management as a requirement for family reunification. As he attempted to engage with Ruth in the intake session, Jim, BSW, noticed that if he mirrored Ruth's body language, he often was able to align with how she was feeling. He matched the position of Ruth's legs while she sat, he mirrored her facial expressions as she spoke and breathed at a similar pace. Whatever Ruth physically expressed, Jim sent back an invisible energetic and physical match. By paying attention to how Ruth's body freely and authentically expressed itself, Jim was able to convey that he was emotionally aligned with her.

VIGNETTE 3.8 NUANCES OF MIRRORING

Luis, a young physical therapist, entered Yasmine's room with his usual enthusiasm and a kind greeting. Yasmine, a Black woman, immediately told him to "knock off the smile". He apologized and changed his facial expression and tone of voice to reflect concern for Yasmine and asked how she was doing. Yasmine said she had no patience for any cheerful, "chirpy" therapist making false promises about her recovery. Luis was able to connect with Yasmine by matching the nuances of her non-verbal communication, and physical therapy then proceeded well. Over the weeks, Yasmine worked hard in her sessions with Luis and shed tears of joy as she recovered her ability to walk.

VIGNETTE 3.9 COMPLEXITIES OF MIRRORING: SỰ PHỨC TẠP CỦA PHẢN CHIẾU

When Hau, a middle-aged Vietnamese woman arrives at the cancer centre, she is asked how she is feeling after hearing the news that her cancer is in remission. Her face lights up, she shakes joyously and declares "fantastic". By listening to the tone of her voice, noticing the joy on her face, and seeing Hau's exuberant energy expressed in how she moves her body, Jessica, an RN, energetically and physically mirrors what she sees. With a broad smile, she claps while stating, "fabulous". As

> *the interview continues, Hau's posture changes. She looks downward, avoiding eye contact, and begins to turn away. Conscious of not wanting to mirror Hau's physical posturing, Jessica instead mirrors her initial energy with an energetic posture of openness, warmth, and possibility. This allows Hau to continue sharing.*

As is highlighted in vignettes 3.7, 3.8, and 3.9, mirroring and matching the tone of voice and posture of a client can build rapport and evoke a connection. At other times, an attuned listener loans their confidence, perhaps both verbally and non-verbally, to an individual who no longer believes in themselves or uses humour to break a pattern of discouragement or defeat. Jessica, in vignette 3.9, shows how artful communication is responsive to each person and to each new situation with a fresh and effective approach. Although there may be some racial or cultural norms to be aware of, there are no formulas for individuals.

Standing versus sitting

Swayden et al. (2012) conducted a randomized controlled study with 120 adult post-operative inpatients admitted for elective spine surgery to compare patient perceptions of the length of interactions, depending on whether the physician stood or sat at the bedside. Even though the actual time the physician spent at the bedside did not change significantly whether they sat or stood, patients with whom the physician sat reported longer consultations, more positive interactions, and a better understanding of their condition by the physician. Although consultations only lasted 60–120 seconds, researchers were amazed that some patients perceived consultations where the physician sat at the bedside as lasting 5–15 minutes. It would appear that physicians who sat next to patients during consultations appeared to be more attuned with their clients than those who stood by the bedside.

Deepening attunement

To deepen awareness of non-verbal communication, listening partners are encouraged to address the non-verbal communication they have noticed in their own interactions with each other, health care providers, family members, friends, and co-workers from diverse backgrounds. What variations have they noticed related to race or culture? What kind of non-verbal communication do they desire in interactions with others? Have they observed their own non-verbal communication on video recordings? If not, can they do so with a listening partner? Laughing off any tension and embarrassment about how we see ourselves on video recordings with a trusted ally can help in enhancing one's ability to be even more flexible and attuned as non-verbal communicators. Table 3.1 offers a variety of listening partnership questions and journal prompts to support the development of presence and

TABLE 3.1 Presence and attunement

Listening and beyond: Dimensions of engaged listening	Questions for dialogue and connection — Each speaker decides on which question(s) they would like to answer	Journal/discussion prompts
Presence Mind free of distractions Not interrupting Allowing for silences (1 minute each way – listener says nothing) ★This is the only listening partnership where the listener says nothing.	Consider your cultural and racial background as you answer these questions: • What were communication patterns like in your family of origin? • Are you more comfortable listening or speaking? • What is it like to allow for silences? • Why do you want to be a health or social care practitioner?	1. What was it like to listen and be listened to for 1 minute without interrupting? 2. Discuss if you would have preferred more or less time and for your partner to say anything? 3. What kind of non-verbal communication did you use? 4. What helps you keep your mind free of distractions when listening? 5. Was culture or race a factor in your experience of listening without interrupting?
Attunement Eye contact Body language Posture and facial expression Fidgeting (2 minutes each way)	What have you noticed about the non-verbal communication of people from different racial and cultural backgrounds? • What have you noticed about your non-verbal communication? Can you sit still, or do you fidget? • What is it like to make eye contact as a listener or a speaker? • Have there been times when you did not feel listened to because of someone's non-verbal behaviour? • Talk about how technology affects non-verbal communication.	6. Was this listening partnership any easier than the first one? 7. Were you conscious of your non-verbal behaviour, as you were the listener? 8. What did your partner do well in terms of non-verbal communication? 9. Would it be useful to practise different facial expressions in front of a mirror or use a video recording to develop more awareness and flexibility? 10. Discuss if you have been able to continue practising not interrupting.

Adapted from: Froehlich, J. (2017), pp 106–107.

attunement. In Chapter 4, we will explore deepening our ability to be present and attuned as we lovingly invite and listen to life narratives.

References

Beckman, H. B., & Frankel, R. M. (1984). The effect of physician behavior on the collection of data. *Annals of Internal Medicine, 101*(5), 692–696. https://doi.org/10.7326/0003-4819-101-5-692

Danczak, A. (2015). British GPs keep going for longer: Is the 12 second interruption history? *British Medical Journal, 351*, h6136. https://doi.org/10.1136/bmj.h6136

Froehlich, J. (2017). Effective communication. In K. Jacobs & N. MacRae (Eds), *Occupational therapy essentials for clinical competence* (3rd ed., pp. 99–132). Thorofare, NJ: SLACK, Inc.

Froehlich, J., Pardue, K., & Dunbar, D. S. (2016). Evaluation of a communication survey and interprofessional education curriculum for undergraduate health professional students. *Health and Interprofessional Practice, 2*(4), eP1082. https://hipe-pub.org/articles/abstract/10.7772/2159-1253.1082/

Jackins, H. (1981). *The art of listening.* Seattle, WA: Rational Island Publishers.

Joos, S. K., Hickam, D. H., Gordon, G. H., & Baker, L. H. (1996). Effects of a physician communication intervention on patient care outcomes. *Journal of General Internal Medicine, 11*(3), 147–155.

Kabat-Zinn, J. (2009). *Wherever you go, there you are: Mindfulness meditation in everyday life.* Boston, MA: Hachette Books.

Marvel, M. K., Epstein, R. M., Flowers, K., & Beckman, H. B. (1999). Soliciting the patient's agenda: Have we improved? *Journal of the American Medical Association, 281*(3), 283–287. https://doi.org/10.1001/jama.281.3.283

Putnam, S. M., Stiles, W. B., Jacob, M. C., & James, S. A. (1988). Teaching the medical interview. *Journal of General Internal Medicine, 3*(1), 38–47. https://doi.org/10.1007/bf02595755

Rhoades, D. R., McFarland, K. F., Finch, W. H., & Johnson, A. O. (2001). Speaking and interruptions during primary care office visits. *Family Medicine, 33*(7), 528–532. https://pubmed.ncbi.nlm.nih.gov/11456245/

Shafir, R. Z. (2003). *The Zen of listening: Mindful communication in the age of distraction.* Wheaton, IL: Quest Books.

Swayden, K. J., Anderson, K. K., Connelly, L. M., Moran, J. S., McMahon, J. K., & Arnold, P. M. (2012). Effect of sitting vs. standing on perception of provider time at bedside: A pilot study. *Patient Education and Counseling, 86*(2), 166–171. https://doi.org/10.1016/j.pec.2011.05.024

4

LOVING AND INVITING LIFE NARRATIVES

Love and caring as health and social care practitioners

VIGNETTE 4.1 COMPASSIONATE COURAGE: NAXARIIS GEESINIMO LEH

Diric, a 25-year-old male Somalian refugee was brought into the ER with a knife wound to his head. During his physical examination, Akira, NP, asked what happened. Diric shared the experience where he and his partner were cornered by a group of men who taunted them by yelling, "Get out of our neighbourhood. You are not wanted here". Diric shared how much shame he felt that he could not protect his partner, who also received a knife wound. Akira responded, "This must be so hard to talk about. Thanks for opening up to me. I appreciate so much you are trusting me with this. By the way, do you mind if I ask you what your name means?" Diric told Akira that his name meant fearless, daring, and bold in Somalian and was a name that was given to male infants who were destined to grow into heroic and courageous men. Akira smiled knowingly as he nodded: "Your parents are wise. That is a perfect name for who you are."

VIGNETTE 4.2 GOING TO THE CHAPEL

Jody, the occupational therapist, has tried many strategies with Annabelle, but none have motivated her to get out of bed. Exasperated, Jody says, "How about if I wear my wedding dress to work tomorrow, will you get out of bed for me then?"

> *Jody wears her wedding dress to the nursing home the next day, and sure enough, Annabelle chuckles as she gets out of bed and engages in occupational therapy interventions related to her self-care.*
>
> *Froehlich, 2017a, p. 134*

Health and social care team members in vignettes 4.1 and 4.2, Akira and Jody, show their caring, empathy, and compassion towards their clients. When we care for others, we show our kindness and concern – our humour and playfulness. When we show empathy, we are able to put ourselves in the shoes of another and understand their perspective and feelings. When we show compassion, we not only empathize with others, but we take action on their behalf. When we show racial and cultural sensitivity, we care within and across racial and cultural lines. We lovingly ask questions to understand the values, beliefs, and practices of people who are different from us (Maier-Lorentz, 2008). Research shows that caring, empathy, and compassion not only improve the health of our clients but also improve the health and wellbeing of the health practitioner (Doty, 2016; Youngson, 2012). Caring for others can reduce harmful stress, boost cellular healing, heighten immune responses, and even turn on protective genes, and increase longevity (Brown & Brown, 2015; Youngson, 2012).

Many health care practitioners find themselves not only caring for their clients and colleagues, but unabashedly "loving" their clients and team members across a multitude of racial and cultural backgrounds. Although the word "love" has many meanings, most people associate "love" with an intense feeling of deep connection. This feeling transcends romantic relationships, strong familial and kinship ties, close friendships, spiritual connections, and healing relationships.

Hardwired for love

Sheri Mitchell (2018), noted Penobscot writer, reminds us that all humans come from a long lineage of love. Young children naturally care for and love each other. As a species, we survived seemingly insurmountable challenges because we loved and cared for one another. Each individual alive today exists because of the love of thousands of people who have come before them. Considering the mounting evidence in the fields of neuroscience, psychology, biology, and economics showing that our health and wellbeing depend on caring and love, it would appear that humans are "hardwired for love". Psychiatrists Thomas Lewis and colleagues (2000) argue that the ancient emotional architecture of the brain is the "key to our lives" and that love is the "life force" that makes us who we are as humans. Developing humans, and mammals as well, develop limbic resonance, the vital capacity to be attuned to each other's inner states, as a foundation for attachment and love. Without love, both the individual and all of society are damaged. And, as our species has survived over many years because of this loving connection to one another, we cannot survive without love.

In a similar vein, author Maia Szalavitz and child psychiatrist Bruce Perry propose that human connection is so essential for our health and wellbeing that "we are indeed born for love" (Szalavitz & Perry, 2010, p. 5). Recently discovered mirror neurons are the neurological foundation for empathy which in turn is the foundation for love. These cells fire when we do something and also fire when we see someone else do the same thing, thus allowing us to feel both the joy and pain of our fellow humans. However, empathy and love only develop in the context of a rich social milieu whereby people learn to be empathic and learn to love. Hence, knowing how to love others is not automatic, and multiple barriers inherent in modern societies, including racial and cultural lines, stand in the way of humans loving and caring for each other. We often fumble our way towards each other – sometimes we connect deeply, and sometimes we miss the mark despite our best attempts.

Satisfaction in love and caring

VIGNETTE 4.3 I HONOUR YOU: 我很荣幸 WǑ HĚN RÓNGXÌNG

Chen worked long hours as a housekeeper at the hospice facility. She treasured many moments of connection with patients who had only a few days or hours to live. Chen found it unbearable to see anyone die alone – this was against every-thing in her Chinese culture that emphasized community. She made sure to take her time cleaning the rooms of people who were near death, so they were not alone. Chen bowed to honour them as they took their last breath.

VIGNETTE 4.4 MEAN GUY MELTS

Carolyn, a home care nurse, volunteered to do a home visit with Ray – an older white man so mean that two of his previous nurses now refused to provide him with care. As Carolyn approached his house, he let his dogs out and said, "Go get her!" The barking dogs rushed against the fence as Carolyn explained she was there to help Ray with his diabetic medications. Ray pulled the dogs aside and grumbled as he allowed Carolyn to assist him with his insulin. After receiving the same treatment on her third visit, Carolyn yelled at Ray, "You know, I am not here for the money. If I were in it for the money, I wouldn't be a nurse. I'm only here because I care about you." With an incredulous look and tears streaming down his face, Ray said, "You care about me?" Carolyn and Ray then formed a caring partnership in sustaining his health.

Despite the challenge of knowing how best to connect with others, one of the most rewarding aspects of being members of the health and social care teams is that we get to express our love and caring in our daily work. We chose to be health and social care practitioners because we knew the difference our empathy, compassion, and love could make in the lives of any person struggling with illness, disease, disability, and disadvantage. As Chen, in vignette 4.3, and Carolyn in vignette 4.4, exemplify, members of the health and social care teams derive tremendous satisfaction in offering our love and caring to those we serve. We find meaning in our work because we notice the profound healing effects of our compassion and love on those we serve. In a report on the "secrets of physician satisfaction", relationships with patients, colleagues, and family were given the highest ratings and prestige associated with the physician role was given the lowest rating (Bogue et al., 2006).

Juxtaposed against the many times when we can notice the effectiveness of our love and care are the challenging interactions when we can't notice that our care and love matter. It is important to remember that we often have blinders on regarding the significance of our caring. When Inova Health System in Northern Virginia implemented a human caring model in their hospitals, patient satisfaction rose by almost 80% in two of their hospitals. Not surprisingly, there was also a statistically significant improvement in nurse satisfaction scores (Drenkard, 2008).

When we struggle to like someone

VIGNETTE 4.5 CHECKING JUDGMENT AT THE DOOR

Jennifer, an experienced physical therapist, worked with a young white woman living in poverty. Martha, after experiencing whiplash from a car accident, had bilateral wrist and foot drop due to conversion disorder. In other words, her physical disability was in her mind. Her paralysis followed no neurological pattern. She was dependent on others for all mobility and self-care needs including toileting and also smoking. Jennifer was aware that she was very judgmental towards this client and found it immensely frustrating to work with Martha. With guidance from her supervisor, she was able to understand that childhood trauma was the basis for Martha's conversion disorder. Physical therapy proceeded well when she was able to separate Martha as a human being from her problems or distresses. Finding compassion within herself, and using a physical rehabilitation approach, Jennifer assisted Martha in regaining complete independence in walking.

Perhaps even more challenging than not being able to notice that our caring matters are times when we find that we simply don't like, let alone love, our clients and/or team members. Fortunately, respect for the worth and dignity of every human is the base that health and social care practitioners stand upon when we can't empathize or notice that we care for or love our clients. We can choose to offer our respect, even when we do not feel that we like a client or team member – especially when we are able to separate people from their behaviours, attitudes, problems, and distresses as demonstrated by Jennifer in vignette 4.5. As Jackins (1993) so eloquently stated, "Every single human being, when the entire situation is taken into account, has always, at every moment, done the very best that he or she could do, and so deserves neither blame nor reproach from anyone, including self" (p. 3).

Remedies for dislike

VIGNETTE 4.6 HEARTS AND HURTS: A HEALING PARTNERSHIP

Tim had an explosive temper and found himself in a court system that deemed him dangerous. He was charged with assault after swinging a bat against a young Black gay man. Chantelle, BSW, initially dreaded the thought of spending time with Tim and did not understand how she would be able to connect with him – a racist, homophobic, elderly white man. She thought a connection could be possible if she remembered that people who hurt others were often hurt themselves. Tim's hurt was revealed when he shared information about his explosive and violent father who pitted Tim against his older brother and who taught Tim that all men, including Black and gay men, were the enemy. To her amazement, Chantelle's dread melted, and she felt compassion as she listened to the hurt in his life story.

VIGNETTE 4.7 WHEN WE ARE TRIGGERED BY CLIENTS

Ella, an occupational therapist, was working on an inpatient psychiatric unit when she met Sean, a white man battling with alcoholism. During a group treatment session, Sean began discussing his threatening actions and feelings towards his two daughters, ages 23 and 16, as well as his wife who he has been married to for 27 years. Ella began feeling anger towards this man because of the way he was describing what he had said and done to these women, but also because she had experienced an alcoholic parent. She knew that Sean had a disease and that she needed to take a deeper look into Sean to learn who he was as a person, separate from the alcoholism and negative behavior and separate from her own experiences with an alcoholic father in order to create a successful treatment plan for this man.
Adapted from Froehlich, 2017a, p. 136

One might argue that there is always a complex, likeable human to be discovered under the layers of behaviours and traits that we find bothersome – especially when we have the time and skills necessary to listen to their stories as Chantelle, in vignette 4.6, demonstrates. When we don't have the time or resources necessary to discover the likeability of a client or team member, we need to be able to vent about people we don't like with a confidential listener. As Ella in vignette 4.7 exemplifies, engaging in identity or transference checks can shed perspective on negative feelings or confusion we might have about another person as we ask ourselves: who does this person or situation remind us of from our past? How are they or the situation similar or different? What is unresolved about our own past that is triggered in this current situation? How can we make a decision to not let our past experiences intrude in the present relationship? It is also important to assess whether or not we can provide optimal care to someone we don't like and seek supervision on whether or not another clinician should work with this client.

Inviting others to share: News and goods, concerns, and life stories

VIGNETTE 4.8 AN UNEXPECTED OUTPOURING

Claire, an occupational therapist, worked on a general medical acute, inpatient unit. She introduced herself to her client, Robert, a white professional, to let him know she would work with him in the afternoon. Robert perceived Claire's kind attention and began right then to talk about his situation. He was a chiropractor who had a son who had been in a car accident and needed extensive rehabilitation. Unable to find life worth living with his disability, his son committed suicide. Robert felt betrayed by his son and shameful that this could have happened to him, a man so knowledgeable about disability. He had never told anyone his son had killed himself prior to this moment with Claire. He cried heavily with Claire, and she gently touched his shoulder and let him cry for a while. She thanked him for sharing his difficult story and said she would be back later. As she was leaving, a nurse came in and Robert said, "That is the best damn occupational therapist I have ever met."

Froehlich, 2017a, p. 137

VIGNETTE 4.9 I HAVE OUTLIVED EVERYONE: חייתי את כולם

Dylan, RN, was tending to the bruised knees of Devorah, an 84-year-old Ashkenazi Jewish widow, who fell while attempting to manoeuvre around her sleeping cat, Ezzy. After obtaining the necessary medical information about Devorah and tending to the physical care of her injury, Dylan asked: "Is there anyone who can escort you home?" Devorah said no, that she lived alone with Ezzy and she had no surviving family. "I have outlived everyone. I never thought I would live this long. I wasn't supposed to." She then proceeded to share her life story, for the first time, as a Jewish woman who survived the Holocaust. With a similar tenderness and attention that she had devoted to Devorah's knee, Dylan listened. By the time Devorah left the hospital, her healing had begun.

We all possess countless untold stories about our life experiences, and our lives go better when key stories are told to a trusted and caring listener. Sometimes, that trusted listener is our health practitioner like Claire and Dylan in vignettes 4.8 and 4.9. Most practitioners listen to pieces of life stories, both long and short, throughout a day's work. It is an act of love to listen deeply to someone's life story – yet one that requires practice and nurturance. One of the best ways to develop our ability to listen to life stories is to exchange life stories with peers from diverse racial and cultural backgrounds.

Although close-ended questions are important for gathering a variety of health-related information (age, living situation, work, etc.), it is open-ended questions that create the space for people to show themselves, their joys, triumphs, challenges, and concerns. Since many people feel overwhelmed, overburdened, disconnected, and frustrated by the challenges and tensions of daily life, inviting listening partners and clients at the beginning of a session to share "What is new and good?" grounds both the listener and the person sharing their story in the reality that life is good; it is wonderful to be alive; and the good in life outweighs the difficulties and discouragement. Inviting clients to share concerns or challenging life narratives after having first shared "news and goods" can foster a positive perspective on problems and trying circumstances. Balancing attention on what is going well with life's challenges can be elicited using prompts such as "joys and concerns", "roses and thorns", "highs and lows", or whatever terminology works for a given client. Despite the almost constant tug between upward and downward trends in our lives and the world around us, it is important to relish instances when clients and ourselves have nothing but positive news to share.

VIGNETTE 4.10 INVITATIONS TO SHARE WHAT IS MOST DIFFICULT: 邀请分享最重要的内容 YĀOQǏNG FĒNXIǍNG ZUÌ ZHÒNGYÀO DE NÈIRÓNG

Ali, an occupational therapist, was working in a hospital when she had a new evaluation on the intensive care unit. Her new patient, Li, was lying in bed with a battered, swollen face, bruised arms, and blood still under her fingernails. The first session was comprised mainly of an interview and a test of standing tolerance.

Ali's caring and compassion created the safety for Li to be very honest and open about her story. She disclosed intimate details about the last night's events and her abusive relationship. Li was born and raised in China and had come to the states for college. She was a full-time student and lived with her boyfriend, unbeknownst to her family back home. She refused to call her parents or friends in the area for help and planned on returning to her apartment after discharge. Ali struggled with her own convictions that Li needed additional help and should leave her abusive relationship. However, Ali was aware that Li's situation had complexities that she did not fully understand, and that Li had the right to autonomy and the freedom to make her own choices. Ali could only offer herself as a caring and compassionate resource and work with the interprofessional team in making appropriate referrals for support around domestic violence.

Adapted from Froehlich, 2017b, pp. 116–117

VIGNETTE 4.11 A SIGN FROM GOD: UN SIGNE DE DIEU

Claudette, an 86-year-old French Canadian Catholic female was being seen in her home by Marie after a mild stroke. Her occupational therapist noted that she was extremely modest about her body in allowing assistance with self-care. Across several occupational therapy visits where her therapist showed her caring and compassion, Claudette discussed the recent loss of her husband and shared that he had been abusive physically and sexually to her and that she had been sexually abused as a child. She also shared proudly that one night when her husband was very drunk, she shaved a cross on his chest. When he awoke, he thought it was a sign from God, and the drinking and abuse stopped for a while.

Froehlich, 2017b, p. 117

VIGNETTE 4.12 RECONCILIATION

Charlotte, a hospice social worker, asked Marvin, her older white hospice client, what was keeping him from sleeping at night. He finally was able to actually open up and say, "I have so much regret. I used to be very close to my daughter. At night when I am awake in bed, I remember a conversation with my daughter when she told me she was lesbian. I was totally disarmed and rejected her. Now I have missed all that time with her over stupid political bias. I can never undo that." Charlotte was able to make a call to the daughter, explain the situation, and ask how she felt about making contact with her father. The daughter was very receptive, so they had a beautiful conversation on FaceTime. Marvin was weeping, and there was mutual forgiveness. The daughter was with her father for the last three days of his life.

Interviews and assessments are opportunities to invite life stories. The more we listen to our client's heartfelt stories as Ali, Marie, and Charlotte did in vignettes 4.10, 4.11, and 4.12, the deeper we connect and the more the healing process becomes possible. Life stories can be told and listened to from many vantage points, particularly from the perspectives of race and culture, to build awareness and appreciation of oneself and diverse individuals, communities, and populations. Our relaxed love, caring, and compassion combined with our inviting presence, and attunement, fuel the outpouring of stories like those of Li, Claudette, and Marvin. Encouraging words such as, "Tell me more" or "What else?", conveyed with a relaxed and caring tone, further allow stories to unfold. Examples of open-ended questions listening partners might ask each other or their clients that transform racial and cultural lines include – "What is your life story as a Black, Brown, or white person? As an immigrant, as a male or a female?" Table 4.1 and Tables C.2 and C.3 in Appendix C provide many additional questions that invite listening partners to share their life stories with a focus on both pleasant memories and challenging experiences across the life span with attention to racial and cultural nuances. Feedback at the end of listening partnerships or practitioner interactions that focus on what the listener did well and one area for improvement will guide the listener in rapidly making improvements.

Life goals, hopes, and dreams

VIGNETTE 4.13 SHE LIT UP LIKE A CHRISTMAS TREE

Janey, a white 4-year-old girl at a center for children with disabilities, had hypoglossia-hypodactylia which presented with the absence of hands and feet. She was a brilliant and determined little girl who was eager to participate in the world by using all kinds of utensils and craft tools. Bilateral activities were extra challenging for Janey, but 6 months into therapy, she expressed with a vehemence that she really wanted to use scissors. With some trial and error, her occupational therapy practitioner, Marie created a custom scissor block, with mounted spring-loaded scissors angled so gravity assisted in cutting. This scissor block enabled Janey to use one residual limb to stabilize the paper and the other to actively cut. When she saw the scissor block and tried it for the first time, Marie said, "She lit up like a Christmas Tree." Despite being a shy girl, she proclaimed to everyone in her class, "Look at me, look at what I can do!" She wanted to cut paper grass for spring baskets for all 8 of her peers.

Froehlich, 2017a, p. 138

> ## VIGNETTE 4.14 RECLAIMING HEALTH: RUNNING FOR HIS LIFE
>
> *Miguel was providing physical therapy to help John, a young Black man, adjust to his new prosthetic leg. John was injured in the Iranian missile strike on a US base in Iraq after the assassination of General Suleimani in January 2020 and spoke bitterly about his lost limb, severe headaches, and problems with flashbacks. He had been very disciplined and health-conscious prior to the accident – he ate well and was an avid runner. Now he found himself addicted to e-cigarettes and other nicotine products to cope. Miguel knew he had a good rapport with John, so he asked if he was open to discussing how to reclaim his health and wellbeing again – to explore quitting the use of nicotine and picking up running again with his new prosthetic leg. John's face revealed a new look of possibility as he affirmed his strong interest in reclaiming his health.*

As Marie and Miguel beautifully demonstrate in vignettes 4.13 and 4.14, the hallmark of the client- and patient-centred practice is inviting our clients or patients to identify and share their goals, hopes, and dreams for health, wellbeing, and a better life and working with them to achieve these goals. As we listen to our clients' narratives, we often explore their goals and wishes for the next few days, weeks, months, and/or years. Caring inquiries offer clients a chance to think about their personal priorities, and to stretch their capacity to want a better life for themselves and for the people and world around them.

A nursing model for inviting concerns, goals, and wishes: Take 5

Nurses Nancy Dorenkott and Ashley Jacobs (2012) developed a unique programme called Take 5 on a paediatric medical-surgical unit where nurses were trained to take 5 minutes at the beginning of each shift to give their undivided attention to each patient and family members, while inviting them to share concerns and goals. After introducing themselves and the plan of care for the shift, they asked what the family would like to happen during the upcoming shift, asked about the family's goals and expectations, and anything they could do to make the hospital stay easier. Nurses were asked to document Taking 5 on client logs and visual reminders of the number 5 were posted throughout units. They found that patient satisfaction, overall assessment, and nursing scores all rose dramatically within less than a year of implementing Take 5. Nurses found renewed job satisfaction in this guided practice of connecting with their patients and families around their concerns, goals, and wishes.

Communicating caring and positive expectations

Showing our caring and high or positive expectations for our clients, while also appreciating that, for some people, simply getting their socks on in the morning

TABLE 4.1 Loving and inviting life narratives

Listening and beyond: Dimensions of engaged listening	Questions for dialogue and connection Each speaker decides on which question(s) they would like to answer	Journal/discussion prompts
Love and caring Build rapport Confidentiality Compassion (3–5 minutes each way)	• Describe experiences with love, caring, rapport building, and compassion with people from diverse racial and cultural backgrounds. • What does the word respect mean to you? Is it possible to respect people you do not like? • What do the words love and caring mean to you? Do caring and love have a place in health or social care? • What does compassion mean to you? Empathy?	1. What went well in this listening partnership? 2. What could have made it even better for both individuals? 3. Discuss if there was an opportunity to allow for silence. 4. What helps build rapport and convey compassion within and across racial and cultural lines?
Inviting life narratives Asking questions: news and goods/concerns and challenges (10+ minutes each way)	• Talk about confidentiality in listening partnerships and other relationships. Share your life experiences from the lens of your racial and cultural background: • What is new and good in your life? • What is hard or challenging in your life right now? Or where do you need a hand? Tell me more.	5. Discuss what it was like to share your life experiences from the lens of your racial and cultural background. 6. What was it like to share news and goods as well as challenges and or/concerns with a listening partner? 7. Reflect upon your use of open- and close-ended questions.
Life stories and life goals (15+ minutes each way)	• Discuss what would increase your comfort level in sharing your life story with people from different racial and cultural backgrounds. • What are some pleasant memories of being a child within your family, neighbourhood, school, church, or community? • What was difficult or challenging in your childhood? • What are some pleasant memories of your adolescence? • What was your favourite activity? What made you laugh and who did you laugh with? Talk about your first job. • What was difficult or challenging about being an adolescent? • Talk about what is great and what was or is challenging about being a young adult and/or adult? • What are your goals, both short- and long-term for the health and wellbeing of yourself, your family, your friends, your community, and the living Earth?	8. What did you learn about yourself by sharing and listening to life stories with each other? Discuss any racial and cultural differences that emerged. 9. Where was the most emotion in this exchange? Were you able to delve into the topic that brought up the most emotion? 10. What was it like to share goals with each other? 11. Discuss the relevance of asking questions to understand key concerns and goals in your future practice. 12. What made listening partnerships on your current concerns, goals, and life stories go well, and what could have made them go even better?

Adapted from: Froehlich, J. (2017b), pp 106–107.

is a large achievement, helps people to move forward on their goals. Each small, short-term success builds towards larger, long-term accomplishments and unleashes a gratifying sense of personal power – particularly when we take action on goals of our own choosing. Imposing goals on others is not only contrary to the essence of client/patient-centred practice, but as the research on motivational interviewing shows, does not result in sustainable health behaviour change.

Table 4.1 guides listening partners in deepening connections as they listen to each others' life narratives from the perspective of their racial and cultural backgrounds. Listening partners may also find that identifying and sharing goals, hopes, and wishes with each other, combined with regular check-ins on their accomplishments, can break the isolation that leaves many of us defeated and discouraged from achieving our goals. Being accountable to a trusted peer or professional for both small and large steps towards reaching our goals is the key to action for many people. When our clients and colleagues notice our depth of caring as we listen to their life stories, hopes and dreams, many feelings may surface. In Chapter 5, we address how to align and respond when the depth of connection evokes a range of feelings.

References

Bogue, R. J., Guarneri, J. G., Reed, M., & Hughes, J. (2006). Secrets of physician satisfaction: Study identifies pressure points and reveals life practices of highly satisfied doctors. *Physician Executive, 32*(6), 30–39.

Brown, S. L., & Brown, R. M. (2015, August). Connecting prosocial behavior to improved physical health: Contributions from the neurobiology of parenting. *Neuroscience and Biobehavioral Reviews, 55*, 1–17. https://doi.org/10.1016/j.neubiorev.2015.04.004

Dorenkott, N., & Jacob, A. (2012). *Take 5: Fairview Hospital* [PowerPoint slides]. https://chcm.com/wp-content/uploads/2013/08/34_Fairview%20Hospital-Cleveland%20Clinic_Dorenkott_Take%205.pdf

Doty, J. R. (2016). The blog: Why kindness heals. *Huffington Post*. www.huffingtonpost.com/james-r-doty-md/why-kindness-heals_b_9082134.html

Drenkard, K.N. (2008). Integrating human caring science into a professional nursing practice model. *Critical Care Nurse Clinician North America, 20*(4), 403–414. https://doi.org/10.1016/j.ccell.2008.08.008

Froehlich, J. (2017a). Therapeutic use of self. In K. Jacobs & N. MacRae (Eds), *Occupational therapy essentials for clinical competence* (3rd ed., pp. 133–147). Thorofare, NJ: SLACK, Inc.

Froehlich, J. (2017b). Effective communication. In K. Jacobs & N. MacRae (Eds), *Occupational therapy essentials for clinical competence* (3rd ed., pp. 99–132). Thorofare, NJ: SLACK, Inc.

Jackins, H. (1993). *Quotes.* Seattle, WA: Rational Island Publishers.

Lewis, T., Amini, F., & Lannon, R. (2000). *A general theory of love.* Manhattan, NY: Random House Publishers.

Maier-Lorentz, M. M. (2008). Transcultural nursing: Its importance in nursing practice. *Journal of Cultural Diversity, 15*(1), 37–43.

Mitchell, S. (2018). *Sacred instructions.* Berkeley, CA: North Atlantic Books.

Szalavitz, M., & Perry, B. D. (2010). *Born for love.* New York: HarperCollins Publishers.

Youngson, R. (2012). *Time to care.* Raglan, New Zealand: RebelHeart Publishers.

5

ALIGNING AND RESPONDING TO EMOTIONS

Humankind: Intelligent, vulnerable, and emotional beings

VIGNETTE 5.1 MUSIC AS THE DOOR TO MY SOUL

Social worker, Shantae, was connecting with Jamal, a 16-year-old African American male via video. Jamal had recently been diagnosed with COVID-19 and shared the possibility he may have infected or killed others unknowingly. He struggled to find the words to express his emotions though his face showed the excruciating pain he was in. Shantae remembered Jamal's love of rap music, it allowed him to express a depth of emotion which was not possible through talking. She asked him if there was a particular song that could express the feelings he had been carrying. "Yeah. Rap is the door into my soul. It's how I experience my world. There is a song called 'Forgiveness' by Toby Mac." Shantae found the song on her cell phone and played it. Jamal's head fell back as he silently wailed while the lyrics were sung. Shantae held up her hands to the video screen, imagining she was holding his face while a tear coursed its way down her chin.

VIGNETTE 5.2 GALES OF LAUGHTER

Vanessa, the physical therapy aide, rang Maura's bell several times before she opened the door a tiny crack. Maura, a middle-aged white woman with an intellectual disability, yelled out, "I am too tired for therapy today." Vanessa asked if she could just stay a few moments and Maura reluctantly opened her door. Knowing

> *Maura was heading right back to bed, Vanessa scooted past her and hopped into her bed so Maura couldn't lie down. Maura shrieked gales of laughter as she swatted Vanessa with a pillow. Therapy then proceeded better than usual.*

Humans are inherently kind and intelligent, and we feel deeply. Our remarkable capacity to think and our extraordinary capacity to feel are strongly interrelated. When we are hurt or distressed, our inherent capacity to think logically and respond flexibly and creatively to the world around us is diminished. According to the psychiatrist and best-selling trauma research author Bessel van der Kolk (2014), when humans experience distress, the emotional centre of the brain, the limbic system, is activated, and it is as if the cerebral cortex, the main thought and control centre of the brain, is "emotionally hijacked". Whether we are in flight, fight, grief, or pain mode, information is no longer received, processed, and stored accurately, and our responses to the world around us may become irrational and/or rigid (Jackins, 1994). For example, who cannot relate to feeling "out of their mind" and unable to think clearly at some point in their life because they felt overwhelming fear, grief, anger, or embarrassment?

Emotional processing and recovery from tension, hurt, and trauma

Most people would agree that a good, hearty laugh or a good cry helps clear our minds – rather than being suppressed or repressed, our emotions are processed. Both Jamal and Maura in vignettes 5.1 and 5.2 were fortunate to have practitioners who intuitively assisted them in releasing grief and tension through tears and laughter. William Frey, a biochemist, studied crying and discovered that emotional tears differ from reflex tears that are shed in response to an irritant – emotional tears carry more protein, potassium, and hormones (Frey et al., 1981). He theorized that emotional tears are a survival mechanism which flushes out chemicals involved with stress or sadness and helps humans start over with a blank slate. In his exploration of crying as one of the distinct features of being human, noted author, journalist, and National Geographic Fellow, Chip Walter (2006), extols the benefits of crying for communicating our deepest selves to each other.

Rosenfeld (2018) explored the scientific evidence for "laughter as the best medicine" and identified the following 11 health benefits of laughter:

- sign of goodwill towards others which keeps us safe
- reduces blood pressure
- laughter yoga decreases blood pressure and cortisol levels
- reduces anxiety and other negative emotions
- immune booster
- natural antidepressant
- improves respiration

- improves cardiovascular system
- calms stress hormones
- relieves pain
- burns calories.

Additionally, Dunbar et al. (2011) found that when social laughter, as opposed to laughing alone, is elicited by watching videos or stage performances, pain thresholds are significantly elevated compared with the control condition. Results suggest that the physical action of laughing with other people generates positive effects by triggering endorphin uptake. Perhaps it is no surprise that laughter is not only good for our physical and emotional wellbeing but also boosts our memory. Bains et al. (2014) conducted a randomized controlled trial and found that humour significantly improved short-term memory in healthy older adults. Similarly, psychologist Mark Beeman found that exposure to laughter-inducing comedy film clips also enhanced creative thinking and problem-solving (Kounios & Beeman, 2015).

Alignment in the recovery process

VIGNETTE 5.3 THE ART OF CREATIVE ALIGNMENT: فن المحاذاة الإبداعية FAN ALMUHADHAT AL'IIBDAEIA

Robert, an RN working with a home health agency, was on his way to do a home visit with Nahla, a young Muslim Moroccan mother and her 7-month-old son, Anouar. He had built trust with Nahla over the past 8 months as a result of providing in-home care for her sick son. When Robert arrived at the home, he saw that a neighbour was yelling at Nahla to "Go back where you came from!" His most elegant, intelligent, and loving response was to move in quickly to stand between Nahla and her neighbour. "Hey Nahla, it is so great to see you. It has been such a long time. Why don't we go inside and talk about how your son is doing?" Robert creatively disarmed the person who was verbally attacking Nahla and provided respite to both her and her son.

VIGNETTE 5.4 DONE-DONE-DONE

Sasha, the physical therapist, entered Carl's room to bring him to the physical therapy gym. Carl, an overweight 70-year-old white Southern man had experienced chronic knee pain for several years and finally had a total knee replacement. He was making slow progress in learning to use a walker instead of his wheelchair. When Sasha invited him to join her in going to the physical therapy gym, Carl refused, stating he was "done with rehab – done-done-done!" Sasha immediately

> stated, "Of course, you're done – who, in your situation, wouldn't feel done?" Carl, disarmed by Sasha's alignment with his feelings, replied, "What the 'F***', what kind of therapist are you?" Sasha replied, "The kind of therapist that isn't done with you!"

As we see in Robert and Sasha's alignment with their clients in vignettes 5.3 and 5.4, the magnificent human mind triumphs best over stress, hurt, and tension when we can release and process emotions in the presence of those with whom we feel safe and connected. Jackins (1994) describes the natural recovery process from hurts as uniquely and inherently human. He extends the outward manifestation of this healing process beyond laughing and crying to include shaking, sweating, raging, yawning, and interested, non-repetitive talking. Although many people find that they can have a good cry or laugh on their own, there are limitations to how fully we can recover our flexible intelligence without a close loving connection with another person.

Variations in using the recovery process

VIGNETTE 5.5 COMMUNAL TEAR-SEEKING: 共同「を求めて KYŌDŌ NAMIDA O MOTOMETE RUI-KATSU

Marco, MSW, was counselling Noriko, a Japanese woman who had recently lost her father. Noriko was raised in a family and in a culture where the expression of emotion was discouraged, and repressing sadness and anger is considered a virtue in Japanese culture. Marco could see that Noriko was working very hard to hold back her tears. No matter how much he encouraged her to allow her tears, Noriko was unable to understand the concept of crying in front of someone who listens. She repeatedly apologized for any tears she shed. In an attempt to normalize the expression of grief, Marco shared with Noriko that in Japan, there are groups of people who gather together at events to watch videos and movie clips of sad events, YouTube memorials for pet cats or dogs – and they bawl together. Why not cry with others who are crying?

Young children around the world naturally seek closeness and comfort when they are stressed or hurt. They expect key allies in their lives to be with them as they express all manner of grief, fear, and distress. Despite some variations in using our inherent recovery process, in general, the outpouring of emotions when we are hurt is inhibited across racial and cultural lines from a young age. Widespread conditioning trains us to keep our feelings "under wraps". Nonetheless, females are inclined to hold onto their capacity to cry more than males (Collier, 2014). With a few exceptions, individuals in more affluent, democratic, and extroverted countries such as the United States tend to report more crying (van Hemert et al., 2011). To counter the strong taboo against crying in Japan, the practice of communal *rui-katsu*, or "tear- seeking" has been developed. Crying clubs support the lovely shedding of tears in connection with others (Shimbun, 2013; St Michel, 2015). As a culturally aware therapist, Marco lovingly introduces Noriko to *rui-katsu* in vignette 5.5.

Health and social care practitioners: Natural allies in healing

VIGNETTE 5.6 TEARS TO HEAL EMBARRASSMENT: TRÄNEN ZU HEILEN

Marie, an occupational therapist, was assisting a German American gentleman with dementia in transitioning to a new residence. He had incontinence and started to cry and stated, "I am so embarrassed, I wet my pants in front of you." Marie shared that it was not his fault and he cried more. She reassured him it is okay to cry, that this is a big change for him.

Adapted from: Froehlich, 2017, p. 111

Despite the conditioning to inhibit our feelings, health care professionals often find that their clients openly show feelings in their presence. The simple gesture of offering our caring attention or compassionate touch may be the catalyst for our clients to show their deepest worries, grief, and fear. Furthermore, when we are aligned with our clients as they express their feelings, we often, wittingly or unwittingly, turn up the volume on their emotional outpourings as described in vignette 5.6 with Marie and her gentlemen client.

Responding to outpouring of emotions

VIGNETTE 5.7 TENDER TEARS OF CONNECTION: عطاء دموع الاتصال EATA' DUMUE ALAITISAL

After Robert shifted the emotional energy of the neighbour who was verbally abusing Nahla in vignette 5.3, he put his attention on inviting Nahla to share. "I can't imagine what you must be feeling right now. I am here for you if you want to share." Nahla immediately felt safe to shake and cry as she recounted how terrified she was for herself and her son. Robert listened lovingly. Later, as he allowed himself to relax in the safety of his car, Robert's body would not stop shaking. He cried tenderly as he remembered the verbal abuse he had experienced from his father.

VIGNETTE 5.8 SWEARING ONE'S WAY TO RECOVERY: JURER SON CHEMIN VERS LA GUÉRISON

As Germaine, a young Franco heritage woman, shared her frustration with her physical therapist Pascal about how painful her exercises were, she began to swear about how difficult it was to sit up in bed. Pascal welcomed her to swear her way to recovery in English or her mother tongue, French.

How does one best respond to outpourings of feelings? The mindful practitioner quickly assesses the situation and decides to either welcome the release and processing of painful emotions or to assist the individual in getting their attention off their distress. There is a time and a place for each response and Chapter 6 addresses the latter. Practitioners, like Robert and Pascal in vignettes 5.7 and 5.8, who support their clients in venting do so because they are keenly aware that this process deepens bonds and creates possibilities for profound healing. Even listening with care and compassion for 2 minutes while someone vents can transform relationships and improve the effectiveness of our care.

Clients, colleagues, and friends alike sense whether or not people have the attention to listen while they vent or express deep emotion. Developing the attention to listen to a client or colleague express deep emotion is an invaluable skill that requires modelling and practice. If you grew up in a family, community, a racial or cultural group where people were able to express feelings freely, you will have more attention when a client needs to vent. If you did not grow up in such a circumstance, you can develop the ability through listening partnerships to listen to others express feelings. The process of taking turns in venting our feelings and listening to each other's grief, embarrassment, fear, tension, resentment, etc. as trusted allies will not only assist in the development of essential communication skills but can regenerate exhausted, careworn practitioners. Additionally, the skill of maintaining mental focus when someone is upset is also cultivated.

Validations

VIGNETTE 5.9 AGAINST ALL ODDS: CONTRA TODAS AS PROBABILIDADES

Chris, BSW, had monthly visits with Pedro, a Brazilian father imprisoned for a mistake that may ultimately steal 6 years of his young life. The relationship they developed enabled each of them to see the goodness in each other. Pedro shared about his daughter and the regrets of not being able to be there for her. He shared how particularly proud he was of being in the men's support group that Chris led. Chris validated him: "How you show up for others in a group is a powerful way to support your daughter as you focus on being the best man that you can be while living within an oppressive penal system. Also, you deserve to feel complete pride in being a good man. Against all odds, you have done your best to keep your dignity and integrity intact while imprisoned."

VIGNETTE 5.10 WARRIOR WOMAN: NAABAAHII CHIKĘ́Ę́H

Ellen is a social worker with Child Protective Services. She was called in to evaluate a young Indigenous mother, Talula, after the department received an anonymous call describing a filthy and dirty baby. Talula was an overwhelmed young single parent of a 2-month-old child; she was doing her best to go to school part-time and work full-time. As Ellen observed Talula connecting with her child, it was evident that Talula loved her child deeply. She also understood that the caller had focused their attention on the less than immaculate child, wearing clothing too large, stained, and with holes. The child's feet were dirty as a result of being freed from being encased in booties. The caller expressed concern about the quality of Talula's mothering and was unable to notice that the baby was also swaddled and bundled close to Talula's beating heart – wrapped and safely protected while comfortably sleeping. After inviting Talula to share what it had been like to be a single parent, Ellen declared: "I am so proud of you. You are quite a warrior mother. I am in your corner. Now, what can I do to support you?"

As they listened with compassion to their clients' heartfelt stories, Chris and Ellen were able to see that Pedro and Talula in vignettes 5.9 and 5.10 were doing their best in extremely difficult situations. Their authentic validations will deepen trust and allow Pedro and Talula to show themselves and their feelings even more fully. Any phrase that shows understanding and awareness of the complexities of any client's given situation, and the reality that they have done their best with what they have been handed, can be deeply validating. Other examples of potentially validating responses might include, "You deserve to feel proud for handling your situation so well", "Nobody should have to endure such …", "That sounds really hard", or "That sucks". Validations can also be offered in phrases that recognize the inherent goodness, caring, and power of the client.

Reflections, summaries, and clarification

VIGNETTE 5.11 NO LONGER ALONE: YA NO ESTOY SOLO

During intake for a women's support group, Betty, a Cuban American whose preferred pronouns are "she" and "her", described to Santelle, MSW, an experience that had led Betty to look for a support group. "My partner, Sara, a trans woman, began to seek exclusive companionship with people in our friends' circle. I would not have minded if she had not excluded me. Sara and I had built a community of loving and supportive straight, trans, non-binary, and lesbian women. Then Sara and our friends turned their backs on me and even began to gossip about me. There is nothing more painful than to have one's community turn its back on you. It is not that I can easily reach out to new people." Santelle reflected: "Thank you for trusting me with what happened and for sharing how painful that betrayal was by Sara. It also sounds like the experience was especially hurtful when you were also rejected by other people in your community who began spreading mistruths and lies about you. And you now feel alone and abandoned. Did I hear you correctly? Thank you so much for reaching out for support. You are no longer alone."

VIGNETTE 5.12 I SEE YOU AND YOUR PEOPLE

Susan, a Chinese NP with the Public Health Department, had been invited to participate in a forum set up to address the health concerns of the community. The community is predominantly Black and working-class with the majority of households being single mothers. One by one, each person shared stories of high blood pressure, depression, obesity, heart disease, and diabetes and how these health challenges directly impacted lives already ravaged by poverty, police violence, drug abuse, unemployment, crime, and anti-Black racism. After listening intently, Susan said: "Let me make sure I understand your key concerns." After summarizing the key points, she sought clarification: "Are you saying that your community is really being 'f****d over' by anti-Black racism that puts your community at a high risk for multiple health problems and you want the authorities to stop flapping their lips and take action now?"

As we listen to our clients' outpourings of thoughts and feelings, it may make sense to reflect back what we have heard as Santelle did with Betty in vignette 5.11. Reflections embody both the content and feelings that are often subtly expressed (Davis & Musolino, 2016). Phrases such as "it sounds like that was awfully difficult for you" or "you seem extremely (angry, frustrated, scared, etc.) by this situation" can enable people to open up further. Susan, in vignette 5.12, uses summaries and clarifications to ensure she has correctly understood key concerns. She uses words that fortify her alignment with the group as a base for moving forward with them. Rollnick et al. (2008) describe summaries used in motivational interviewing as the bouquets that we hand our clients. A well-delivered summary breaks down feelings of isolation and represents the alignment of two minds in solving health problems together. Acknowledging that we cannot fully put ourselves in the shoes

TABLE 5.1 Aligning and responding to emotions

Listening and beyond: Dimensions of engaged listening	*Questions for dialogue and connection* Each speaker decides on which question(s) they would like to answer	*Journal/discussion prompts*
Validation **Restatement** **Clarification** **Summaries** **Reflection** **Mental focus** **Supporting emotional release** (15+ minutes each way)	What is it like to align or connect with people within and across racial and cultural lines no matter how they present or how they are feeling? • How can you tell when you are aligned or not aligned with someone? • Talk about times when you felt validated or invalidated by a listener. • Talk about times when you offered your validation to someone. • Share what it is like to use restatement, clarification, validation, and summaries in difficult conversations. • Describe emotional expression in your family. Were there any gender differences in the expression of emotion? • Discuss any cultural or racial differences you have noticed in the expression of emotion. • What do you currently do when you feel upset? Is there anyone you can turn to when you need to cry? • What do you anticipate it will be like to listen to future clients who share painful emotions?	1. Reflect upon how to strengthen your alignment with your listening partner or partners. 2. Identify your strengths and areas for improvement in using validation, restatement, clarification, and summaries as a listener. 3. Summarize what your listening partner shares and give each other feedback. 4. With whom do you feel comfortable venting your emotions? What would it take to feel comfortable venting to a listening partner? 5. What have you noticed about how you think and feel when you have had a chance to laugh, cry, shake, or rage? Have you been able to listen to someone when they cried hard? 6. Discuss what it is like to maintain mental focus when someone is upset. Can you do this when someone is upset with you? 7. Discuss which emotions are the easiest for you to listen to. 8. Are you able to stay in roles as a listener and speaker in your listening partnerships?

Adapted from: Froehlich, J. (2017), pp 106–107.

of someone with a particular illness, disability, life circumstance, or racial and cultural background but wish to understand their experiences opens the door to deeper connection and healing.

Aligning with and artfully responding to our clients as they share their deepest worries, fears, tensions, and grief facilitates tremendous healing. The reader will find many questions and journal prompts in Table 5.1 that support deeper alignment with listening partners, friends, colleagues, and ultimately with future clients. In Chapter 6, we explore the many nuances of communication that lift spirits and break the discouragement and despair that plague many clients and practitioners alike.

References

Bains, G. S., Berk, L. S., Daher, N., Lohman, E., Schwab, E., Petrofsky, J., & Deshpande, P. (2014, Spring). The effect of humor on short-term memory in older adults: A new component for whole-person wellness. *Advances in Mind Body Medicine, 28*(2),16–24.

Collier, L. (2014, February). Why we cry: New research is opening eyes to the psychology of tears. *Monitor on Psychology, 45*(2), 47. www.apa.org/monitor/2014/02/cry

Davis, C. M., & Musolino, G. M. (2016). *Patient practitioner interaction* (6th ed.). Thorofare, NJ: SLACK, Inc.

Dunbar, R. I. M., Baron, R., Frangou, A., Pearce, E., van Leeuwen, E. J. C., Stow, J., … van Vugt, M. (2011). Social laughter is correlated with an elevated pain threshold. *Proceedings of the Royal Society: Biological Sciences, 279*(1731), 1161–1167. https://doi.org/10.1098/rspb.2011.1373

Frey, W. H., Desota-Johnson, D., Hoffman, C., & McCall, J. T. (1981). Effect of stimulus on the chemical composition of human tears. *American Journal of Ophthalmology, 924*, 559–567. https://doi.org/10.1016/0002-9394(81)90651-6

Froehlich, J. (2017). Effective communication. In K. Jacobs & N. MacRae (Eds), *Occupational therapy essentials for clinical competence* (3rd ed., pp. 99–132). Thorofare, NJ: SLACK, Inc.

Jackins, H. (1994). *The human side of human beings*. Seattle, WA: Rational Island Publishers.

Kounios, J., & Beeman, M. (2015). *The eureka factor: Aha moments, creative insight and the brain*. Manhattan, NY: Random House.

Rollnick, S., Miller, W. R., & Butler, C. (2008). *Motivational interviewing in health care: Helping patients change behavior*. New York: The Guilford Press.

Rosenfeld, J. (2018, April 11). 11 scientific benefits of having a laugh. Mental Floss: Science. http://mentalfloss.com/article/539632/scientific-benefits-having-laugh

Shimbun, C. (2013, June). Participants ease stress level at crying events. *The Japan Times*. www.japantimes.co.jp/news/2013/06/22/national/participants-ease-stress-levels-at-crying-events/#.XIyYtRNKh0u

St Michel, P. (2015, May). Crying it out in Japan. *The Atlantic*. www.theatlantic.com/magazine/archive/2015/05/crying-it-out-in-japan/389528/

Van der Kolk, B. A. (2014). *The body keeps the score: Brain, mind, and body in the healing of trauma*. New York: Viking.

Van Hemert, D. A., van de Vijver, F. J. R., & Vingerhoets, A. J. J. M. (2011). Culture and crying: Prevalence and gender differences. *Cross-Cultural Research, 45*(4), 399–431. https://doi.org/10.1177/1069397111404519

Walter, C. (2006). Why do we cry? *Scientific American Mind, 17*(6), 44–51.

6

LIFTING SPIRITS

Lifting spirits in others and ourselves

VIGNETTE 6.1 DANCING OUT OF REHAB: A GO GLADI WAY A DANCE FROM DIS REHAB PLACE GO NA OSE

As an occupational therapist, I (Patricia) use all kinds of musical genres to inspire my clients to do dishes, to get dressed, to manage a budget, to do exercise. One lady's goal was to dance out of the rehabilitation facility. We did her home evaluation and it turns out she was an undercover cop from Chicago, and she still had her uniform. We brought the uniform to the hospital, and on her discharge date, she put on her uniform and danced out of the hospital. She had surgery and needed to come back, so the next time we did a home evaluation, we came back with another outfit – an African gown. She danced out of rehab with an African gown. For Christmas, there were a couple of African patients and African aides and nurses, so I played songs from Sierra Leone and Liberia and we all started dancing on the unit. People were uplifted.

Whether our clients are ravaged by disease, physical and emotional injury, adapting to lost limbs, undergoing routine but anxiety-provoking procedures, caring for a new baby, shattered by racism or poverty, health care providers experience daily and important opportunities to lift spirits. We do this by offering our hopefulness in the face of discouragement, humour to ease anxiety and embarrassment, and compassionate touch to alleviate pain, isolation, and despair – whenever we can. Like Patricia in vignette 6.1, sometimes we help our clients get their attention off their distress and onto noticing the beauty of the world around them and within them-selves through song, dance, and celebration. Redirection, especially when combined with skilful guidance, can lift spirits when a client has lost focus and is encouraged to put attention on their priorities at the moment. Sharing information and advice that is attuned to a client's level of understanding and readiness for change may be just what is needed to accelerate the healing journey. All this is most possible when our own spirits are lifted by each other as members of health teams, listening part-ners, or trusted peers. Exchanging confidential venting with those who are compas-sionately present and who care for us can fuel careworn practitioners.

Hope

VIGNETTE 6.2 HALLELUJAH – I AM STILL ALIVE!

Tyson, an NP, arrived for his morning rounds at the residential care facility with a heavy heart from years as a nurse. He noticed Charles, a 90-year-old resident who had survived the coronavirus, sitting up in his bed smiling. Tyson commented that he seemed pleased with himself. Charles revealed, "Every morning, no matter what, I start my day by noticing my eyes are open. I think this must mean I am still alive. I feel my heart pounding in my chest and my lungs expand as I breathe. More proof, I am still alive. How grateful I am to be able to notice I am alive. One more precious day alive as a Black man in this world. If I can notice I am alive, I can then notice there is hope. I can then access the courage to keep going. Because if hope dies, my vitality does as well. So instead, I choose every day to notice when I wake up, I am alive – even more so now I can beat that damn virus." A load lifted off Tyson's heart as well.

How do we find hope in a difficult world? Some people are hopeful by decision – they view hope as a discipline that they will actively choose in the defiance of hopelessness. For others, like Charles in vignette 6.2, it is a spiritual dimension of life, a daily practice of responding to the world from the perspective that we can greet our future with inspired anticipation. Others find that hope is the ability to see what is possible in the face of impossibility. For many, taking positive action in the world, particularly in concert with others, clears the clouds of discouragement and generates hope. Hope then fuels more action. The unceasing efforts of humans to seek solutions to seemingly impossible problems would suggest there is a strong reciprocal and synergistic relationship between hope – as a discipline, spiritual prac-tice, or ability to see possibilities – and action as the genesis for hope. From our deep connection to one another, we are reminded of what is possible and can then be inspired to take empowering action steps.

Problems we encounter as health professionals often feel overwhelming. Yet col-lectively, health practitioners are unstoppable. There is no limit to our creativity and innovation to improve human health and wellness. Hope as a discipline is rewarded, reinforced, and buttressed by both our actions and our loving connections as we face even the most trying circumstances. Small winnable victories provide psychological momentum and hope for even larger victories. Hope and loving connections guide us to view mistakes as opportunities for new strategies, new connections, and reframing what is most important and what is possible.

Hope is closely related to a fundamental belief in the human capacity for growth and change. Psychiatric rehabilitation literature emphasizes the significance of believing in the ability of people with mental health and substance abuse problems to recover (Anthony, 1993; Anthony et al., 2002). The recovery perspective, which assumes that new meaning and hope can be found even in the face of catastrophe, can be a foundation for our interactions with discouraged and defeated clients, colleagues, or ourselves in a variety of health care settings.

Humour

VIGNETTE 6.3 MAH-JONGG ANYONE?

Julia, a mental health occupational therapist, was skilled in incorporating laughter and play into her work with clients. She particularly enjoyed Mah-Jongg, a tile-based game that originated in China. Julia also knew that Mah-Jongg had been a favourite pastime of a client, Esther, a middle-aged Jewish woman who had lost all interest in the game after the recent loss of her sister, Sidell. Julia encouraged Esther to share her memories of playing Mah-Jongg with Sidell and the other Jewish women in her neighbourhood. Esther shared how Mah-Jongg had become communal entertainment where opportunities to socialize were created and life-long friendships developed. "Every week we got to find out and share what was happening in each of our lives – the good and the challenging. And most importantly, we had a chance to love, feel joy, tease each other and laugh so hard that our teeth hurt. Any invitation to play Mah-Jongg was pure fun and a time to take a break from the hardness of our lives. Want to play?"

VIGNETTE 6.4 HAIR, BELLY, AND TEETH: THE PERFECT TRIFECTA: 头发，腹部和牙齿：完美的三连冠 TÓUFÀ, FÙBÙ HÉ YÁCHǏ: WÁNMĚI DE SĀN LIÁN GUĀN

Madeleine, a social worker, worked with Wenjing, a woman from China who lived alone in a small apartment. She had been diagnosed with terminal cancer, and the interpreter and the chaplain were with Madeleine to gather background information. When Wenjing and Madeleine looked at each other, they smiled awkwardly.

Both had a twinkle in their eye and started to giggle. As Wenjing's smile grew, she covered her mouth and said to the interpreter, "I hope they do not laugh at me because I have no teeth." Madeleine said through the interpreter, "Tell her I hope no one laughs at me because of my big belly", and she patted her belly. Wenjing started laughing, and then the chaplain said, "I hope no one laughs at me because I have no hair" and everyone laughed, including the interpreter. Wenjing would touch her mouth, then pat Madeleine's belly, and then tap the chaplain's hair while giggling. During their interview about her life story, Wenjing disclosed that when she lived in China, she was very poor and had one son, a biracial child who was left on her doorstep. She was shunned in her community and called "monkey" for having a biracial child and for being poor. As she noticed the compassion in Madeleine's eyes, Wenjing said, "I can tell you see me as fully human." Madeleine delighted in the melting of cultural and language barriers as the two women connected.

Of the many generous gifts bestowed on humanity by the universe, perhaps humour is one of the greatest. Our capacity to find humour in each other, in ourselves, and in the human situation generates connection, reframes hopelessness, and lifts spirits in the direst of situations. Many health practitioners, like Julia in vignette 6.3 and Madeleine in vignette 6.4, naturally infuse comic relief into their practice to help themselves and their clients cope with the tragic and impossible situations we face. Others benefit from deepening their awareness of antecedents to laughter so they can amplify their presence. Was it something the client said or did, or was it something the practitioner said or did, that stimulated laughter to flow? Was it a tone of voice or facial expression? Our analytical minds, in playing detective when someone is laughing, can rise to new levels of fostering humour and playfulness. Recognizing that enhancing laughter enhances and accelerates healing and decreases pain, Patch Adams, a medical doctor and a clown established the Gesundheit! Institute to train health professionals around the world in the art of laughter, clowning, and creativity as practitioners, and all are welcome to join his cadre (Adams & Mylander, 1993).

Aware touch and physical closeness

VIGNETTE 6.5 NO LIMITS TO CLOSENESS: NESSUN LIMITE ALLA VICINANZA

What was most upsetting for Anthony, 94, the husband of Aurora, 92, was the complete inability to be physically close to her. They were a tactile and physically expressive couple. Though he tested negative for the COVID-19 virus, he was in a state of anguish as he accepted that being close to Aurora was not wise. Her hospitalization presented a unique and welcome challenge for Anthony in that he knew her healing would be enhanced by her physical connection to him and his loving touch. He communicated this to Robert, the CNA assigned to her for daily care. They formed a partnership to transform the window outside Aurora's room into a chance to reach for one another and experience closeness through the glass as they smiled and touched through the glass. Anthony also created a virtual connection to her with visual reminders of his loving touch. The window became the template for healing reminders of Anthony's connection with her – pictures that included his outstretched arms reaching for hers, his wedding band twinkling on his finger, his hands in prayer, and his mouth in a playful pucker. Every morning, Aurora woke to his loving presence, and she possessed his visual reminders when he was not able to be at her window.

VIGNETTE 6.6 HIGH-FIVES AND FIST-BUMPS

Pre-COVID 19, Eric, a Black BSW, was adept at using touch in an intentional and strategic way to enhance a sense of connection with his clients. The young Black boys were often from communities where male role models were lacking. Hyper-masculinity, with its exaggerated stereotypical male ways of behaving that emphasized physical toughness, aggressiveness, and dominant sexual prowess, was reinforced and rewarded. These young boys were also socialized to believe that physical touch and closeness were effeminate or gay. Eric had learned that touch, when used with awareness and with the intention of healing, could provide physical expressions of reassurance, connection, and celebration. Eric's knowledge of when to put his hand on their shoulder was developed from an awareness of when his client needed to feel safe and to know he was okay, A high-five was given whenever clients earned a hard-fought grade on a report card and as a way of acknowledging them. Fist-bumps were a celebration whenever they experienced a first-cast in their first play, were chosen for their first team or got their first date, etc. Eric became their physical reminder of love, encouragement, comfort, and validation.

While assisting a frail client in locomoting with pride and dignity from the bed to the toilet, or searching for a point of pain and offering healing touch to an inflamed shoulder, or debriding a burn wound with skill and care, or sitting close and consoling a father who has lost a child, health and social care practitioners are often moved to transcend racial and cultural lines as we offer our loving touch and closeness. Keltner (2010) describes touch as fundamental to human communication, bonding, and health. Touch is our primary language of compassion, and both Robert and Eric in vignettes 6.5 and 6.6 are well aware of the significance of touch.

While non-human primates spend about 10–20% of their waking day grooming each other (Dunbar, 2010), there is notable variation in human touch and physical closeness across racial and cultural groups. To the detriment of their wellbeing, some humans go for long periods with no touch or caring contact, especially now in the coronavirus pandemic.

Cultural differences around touch

The seminal work of Hall (1966), broadly grouped cultures into *contact* cultures and *non-contact* cultures. *Contact* cultures (Southern Europeans, Latina Americans, and Arabs) were assumed to use closer interpersonal distances and engage in more touching than people in *non-contact* cultures (North American, Northern Europe, and Asian populations). In a cross-cultural analysis of 8,943 participants across 42 countries, Sorokowska et al. (2017) found that people living in warmer regions do tend to use closer interpersonal distances and display more physical contact with each other. They also found that younger people engaged in more physical contact, and women tended to prefer greater distance in social and personal interactions with strangers. Provasi (2012) noted that greetings in warmer climates often involve kissing on the cheek, and people who barely know each other may touch each other on the arm or shoulder during conversations. In cooler climates, any touch from a stranger may be offensive. Within the Muslim culture, men and women cannot touch in public, yet two women or two men might walk arm in arm (Mastrorosa, 2019). Since the appropriateness of touching varies by culture and is now distorted for all humans in the coronavirus pandemic, health and social care practitioners will need continually to learn norms regarding touch for different racial and cultural groups. Despite notable differences in touch across cultures, Suvilehto et al. (2019) found that across cultures, the stronger the emotional bond, the more touching is allowed.

Making mistakes around touch

VIGNETTE 6.7 THE VOID OF PHYSICAL TOUCH

Leyla, a 45-year-old white nurse's assistant, was in a marriage that was void of emotional and physical closeness. She chose to spend much of her life working long hours and asking for more and more moments of human connection in the workplace to avoid the painful aloneness of her marriage. Leyla was vulnerable to seeking friendships with patients. Physical touch was especially enticing, and Leyla sought out opportunities to feel physical aliveness with patients who often lacked human connection in their own personal lives. It was only when Leyla learned from her supervisor that a client complained about her excessive hugs that she was able to put her attention on this void within her life. Her need for human connection was what was compelling her to seek out the patients' touch and friendships and to replace the lack of intimacy in her marriage. It was only through marriage counselling that she learned how to heal her marriage and her physical void.

Our human body houses our life experiences – our joys and triumphs, our pain and sorrow, our courage and discouragement, and our racial and cultural identities. Signs of the love we have given and received, our hard work and generosity, our delight, and pleasure in life along with our full range of experiences as members of racial and cultural groups will be visibly and invisibly etched on our bodies. All practitioners need to practise safe physical contact and use appropriate precautions in their work environments. Additionally, being fully present, attuned to non-verbal and verbal communication, and on the path to awareness of racial and cultural similarities and differences around closeness and touch are essential prerequisites for practitioners to effectively offer physical closeness and our healing touch.

Making mistakes as we learn to offer our touch and closeness to people from diverse racial and cultural backgrounds is natural. Many of us struggle to figure out how to be close to others in the pandemic and make mistakes. We may initiate physical closeness with a client who shuns close contact for personal, medical, or cultural reasons; or we may refrain from touching a client who is screaming inside for a reassuring hand on their shoulder as they face an unbearable loss or overwhelming pain. Sometimes we will ask before we touch a client – at other times our loving intelligence will guide us to simply take someone's gloved hand in our gloved hand to show our caring. Sometimes, as is the case with Leyla in vignette 6.7, we seek touch with our clients because we lack touch in our own lives.

Exploring experiences with touch and closeness in our own lives will inform our use of touch as health practitioners. What were touch and closeness like in our families of origin? How have we grown in using touch and closeness as health practitioners? What racial and cultural factors have we noticed in relation to touch? What are our intentions in offering touch to others? What are our goals for becoming increasingly sensitive, aware, and flexible in showing our care through touch?

Attention off distress, redirection, and celebrating the present

VIGNETTE 6.8 HOUSING FIRST

Kamala, an African heritage mother of three young children, had recently received an eviction notice that was not completely unexpected. There were months of wondering about the probability of homelessness which she had escaped many years ago. While homeless, Kamala had been victimized by a man who raped her. As she shared her story with Rhonda, the MSW, Kamala was overcome with terror and powerlessness, overshadowing the urgency of her need to find a safe place for her family. Rhonda listened with compassion: "I appreciate your courage to have survived the horrible experience of a man who violated the safety of your body and of your spirit. I also appreciate your need to find a safe place for your family. Both are equally important. Would you be open to my assisting you today with finding safe and secure housing for your family and referring you for ongoing support as you heal from the experience of the rape?"

VIGNETTE 6.9 PLAYING THROUGH THE PAIN: اللعب من خلال الألم ALLAEB MIN KHILAL AL'ALM

Marlena, an 8-year-old Lebanese American, was diagnosed with complex regional pain syndrome and could not tolerate any weight bearing or touch on her left leg. Sophia, the physical therapist, gently but firmly insisted that Marlena engage in playing a game of catch and also move through an obstacle course so she would use her affected leg. Sophia was able to skilfully direct Marlena's attention off the excruciating pain in her leg as she engaged in games that forced her to bear weight on her left leg. Ultimately, after a month of bi-weekly physical therapy, Marlena recovered her full ability to use her left leg.

While there is a time and place for supporting our clients in expressing their frustrations, tensions, griefs, and fears, health and social care practitioners spend many of their working hours creatively assisting clients in getting their attention off their distress and in being more able to function in the present. In our first vignette of this chapter, 6.1, Patricia shares several examples of celebrating present moments with her clients and colleagues using music and dance. Both Rhonda and Sophia, in vignettes 6.8 and 6.9, artfully assist discouraged clients in focusing their attention off their distress and onto what needs doing in the present.

On the other hand, the practitioner who is not comfortable with emotional release may err on the side of too quickly redirecting a client's attention away from emotions that need to be released. Some clients may adamantly refuse to focus their attention off their distress or to be redirected until they can tell that their emotional concerns have been heard and understood. Other clients may be terribly uncomfortable with the expression of feelings in the presence of their health practitioner and may welcome redirection and interactions that focus attention off their distress. A client with a wandering mind may also appreciate being redirected to what is most important, and every health practitioner needs to know how to redirect clients and colleagues when *time is up*.

Besides the many therapeutic interventions that practitioners use to support distressed clients in focusing their attention on the present, a few simple yet effective techniques are noted below:

- When *time is up* in a session, simply saying "just because of time, we must conclude our session" conveys that more time might be warranted but cannot be given right now. Using a timer to signal that *time is up* can help a practitioner focus what a client is saying rather than double-checking a clock or watch.
- Asking a client to attend to sharing several sights, sounds, and smells in the world around them (e.g. four blue things in the room or something outside that captures their attention) or to share something they are looking forward to can shift their attention onto the present. Simple word games (creating a nonsense sentence out of the letters in a word – e.g. Flower = fun lovers often wake every rooster) or math games (counting backwards by 3s from 100 or a phone number backwards) may help people without math or word phobias to get their attention off their distress. Guidance from clients about what helps them get their attention off their distress is always helpful.
- When a client's disclosures have lost focus, appreciating the client for sharing before returning attention to priorities may aid the transition.

Sharing ideas and advice

VIGNETTE 6.10 JUDGMENT NO MORE

Robert, the 7-year-old son of Christian Science parents, showed up in the emergency room with his mother, Barbara, an African American woman, cradling him – he had a broken thumb. After tending to the broken bone and placing a splint on the thumb, Cindy, NP, gave the mother a prescription for pain meds. Barbara disclosed that she was not interested in medicine for her child and she would be seeking healing from a Christian Science practitioner. Cindy responded, "Would you be open to some of my thoughts that I can add to what you have figured out already?" Barbara responded, "I am only open to hearing what you have to say if you do not reprimand me about my parenting; if you can stay away from judging me for believing in prayers that heal and if you do not say I am a bad parent, I will be open to what you have to share." Cindy stated that she could honour Barbara by sharing in that way.

VIGNETTE 6.11 ABSOLUTION AND PENANCE

Raquel, a white woman, was finding urinary incontinence an increasing problem in her life post-menopause. She was able to laugh with Winona, her physical therapist, about the embarrassing nature of her problem and some of the assessments, interventions, and prescribed home exercises. She was not able to motivate herself to complete the pelvic floor exercises prescribed by Winona once she was discharged from physical therapy. Within a month, in her urgency to reach the bathroom at night-time, she tripped over her dog and sustained a sprain to her left ankle. Winona was the only practitioner with whom Raquel felt comfortable disclosing that her urinary incontinence was the reason for her fall. Since both women were Catholics, Winona listened to Raquel's confession, jokingly absolved her for her sins, celebrated that the dog was not injured and delivered the penance that Raquel would from now on engage in her pelvic floor exercises regularly. Raquel agreed.

To give or not to give advice or information? Many clients are eager or in some cases desperate for ideas, suggestions, and advice from health practitioners to relieve pain and suffering, to improve health and wellbeing. At the same time, there is probably not a health practitioner or human being who has not shared information or advice with a client or friend to no avail. As we know from motivational interviewing (Rollnick et al., 2008), unless someone is ready to hear and accept our advice, we waste precious time sharing our suggestions. As we see illustrated by Cindy and Winona in vignettes 6.10 and 6.11, when listening and caring are at the base of a relationship, advice can more readily be heard and acted upon.

How can we tell when a client is ready to hear advice? Although some practitioners intuitively know when a client is ready for our words of wisdom, others miss the mark in assuming that a client is ready to adopt our suggestions for new habits and self-care routines or in assuming that a client is not ready for change. Understanding the stages of health behaviour change (pre-contemplation, contemplation, preparation, action, and maintenance) and how to skilfully ask questions to identify these stages in our clients lay the groundwork for compassionate and engaged listening as the path towards change (Prochaska & DiClemente, 1983; Prochaska et al., 1992).

Some clients will find their inner drive to make changes simply because we have asked the right questions, listened, and offered our love and belief in their ability to change. Once we have established a strong relationship, humbly asking permission to share our ideas and advice will in some cases be the perfect strategy to assist change – particularly when our information and advice is in a plain language that considers racial and cultural nuances and is linguistically appropriate (LaRochelle & Karpinski, 2016).

Lifting spirits in teams: Confidential venting with integrity

VIGNETTE 6.12 MUTUAL AID: 공제 GONGJE

Bethany, a white nurse, is at her wit's end as she copes with the many recent deaths in the ICU. Her colleague Yeon, a Korean woman, notices the despair in her eyes and says it is okay to take some time. Bethany apologizes as she sobs for a few moments while Yeon offers her loving and steady attention. Yeon reminds Bethany that it is good to get it all out so she can go forward. When her cries subside, Yeon asks what she is looking forward to and Bethany talks about taking a warm bath when she gets home. Yeon then asks if she can vent too and Bethany gladly listens as Yeon shakes and sweats a little as she shares about a client hatefully stating that Asians are to blame for the coronavirus while refusing to be cared for by Yeon. As Bethany shares her indignation and invites Yeon to tell her more, Yeon is able to talk and shake about other experiences of mistreatment as an Asian person. When Bethany asks what she can do to help Yeon, Yeon says that for now, she just needs to know she has someone who can listen to her and keep confidentiality. Bethany agrees, and when Yeon is ready to get back to work asks her what she is looking forward to. Yeon says she looks forward to relaxing a little more now she knows she has an ally on her side.

VIGNETTE 6.13 UNITED AGAINST GENOCIDE: ÉNSKA əˈGEɪNST ˈʤɛNəSAID

Vivian, a Mohawk PA, and Michael, an African Heritage nurse, are on break from double shifts in the ICU. They share grief and frustration about how badly the coronavirus is affecting Black and Brown people. Vivian shares a photoshopped image of a Native American Chief wearing a traditional feathered headdress along with a full facial mask – military hazmat style. The caption reads "Fighting viruses, pandemics, and invasive species since 1492". Vivian and Michael laugh and agree it is about time that white people understood that large numbers of people dying is nothing new for Brown- and Black-skinned people around the world. They concur that they love many white people, but sure wish more of them had a clue about racism and genocide.

Our daily work lives as health practitioners, students, and workers are fraught with stress and frustration. Confidential venting to trusted peers enables many health practitioners to handle highly stressful situations and then move on to be more fully present with the next patient, client, or situation. How do we vent to each other with integrity when we are triggered by the behaviour, emotions, and attitudes of others and at the same time remember the integrity of our clients, patients, and colleagues?

Choosing someone whom we know can keep confidentiality and asking if they have a few minutes to listen to us vent can be enormously helpful. We may even make an agreement to exchange several minutes of listening if they also have something to vent about. Reminders about confidentiality even to people who generally keep confidentiality are sometimes warranted because there is a pull to share hard stories with others outside of listening exchanges. Acknowledging that we are triggered and releasing our feelings by talking, shedding a few angry words or tears, or laughing with someone we feel connected to will allow us to see difficult

TABLE 6.1 Lifting spirits

Listening and beyond: Dimensions of engaged listening	Questions for dialogue and connection Each speaker decides on which question(s) they would like to answer	Journal/discussion prompts
Hopefulness **Humour** **Touch** **Redirection** **Attention off distress** **Advice/information** (15+ minutes each way)	Share experiences from within and across racial and cultural lines. • What makes you hopeful when you are discouraged? • What kind of humour lifts your spirits? Can you help others laugh to lift their spirits? • Does culture or race play a role in humour in your life? • Talk about the role of touch in health and social care and your comfort level with touch within and across racial and cultural groups. • Share a time when you were redirected or wanted to redirect someone and were or were not successful. • Talk about times when you helped someone, or they helped you get your attention off your distress. • Talk about times when you were given advice or information and it was or was not effective or welcome.	1. Discuss what it is like to maintain hopefulness and use humour and touch when listening. 2. What have you learned about adapting touch in COVID-19? 3. In your future practice, what do you anticipate it will be like to redirect or help clients from diverse racial and cultural backgrounds to get their attention off their distress and to celebrate the present? 4. Explore situations where it may be hard to redirect a client.

Adapted from: Froehlich, J. (2017), pp 106–107.

situations more clearly and decide our next steps. Were we treated unfairly? Do we need to confront someone or seek assistance in doing so? Or, is there something we did that needs to change? Perhaps, rather than blaming the individual towards whom we have less than positive feelings, we need to explore our participation in the problem. Or, is the problem more about stress, pressure, and insufficient resources in the health care system rather than individual flaws?

The health practitioners in vignettes 6.12 and 6.13 provide us with excellent examples of mutually supportive venting that does not denigrate anyone. Only through an agreement with others, to uphold integrity in our venting, can we effectively seek solutions to difficult interpersonal situations that arise in health care and life. Confidential venting with trusted allies can be an important fuel that rejuvenates us in our journey as healers and members of interprofessional teams. There are many additional complex dimensions to interprofessional health care team communication and team functioning that are addressed in Chapter 7. Be sure to exchange listening using the partnership questions on lifting spirits noted in Table 6.1 and explore the journal prompts before moving on to Chapter 7.

References

Adams, P., & Mylander, M. (1993). *Gesundheit! Bringing good health to you, the medical system, and society through physician service, complementary therapies, humor and joy.* Rochester, VT: Healing Arts Press.

Anthony, W., Cohen, M., Farkas, M., & Gagne, C. (2002). *Psychiatric rehabilitation* (2nd ed.). Boston, MA: Center for Psychiatric Rehabilitation.

Anthony, W. A. (1993). Recovery from mental illness: The guiding vision of the mental health service system in the 1990s. *Psychosocial Rehabilitation Journal, 16*(4), 11–23. https://doi.org/10.1037/h0095655

Dunbar, R. I. M. (2010). The social role of touch in humans and primates: Behavioural function and neurobiological mechanisms. *Neuroscience and Biobehavioral Reviews, 34*, 260–268. https://doi.org/10.1016/j.neubiorev.2008.07.001

Froehlich, J. (2017). Effective communication. In K. Jacobs, & N. MacRae (Eds), *Occupational therapy essentials for clinical competence* (3rd ed., pp. 99–132).

Hall, E. T. (1966). *The hidden dimension.* New York: Doubleday.

Keltner, D. (2010, September 29). Hands on research: The science of touch. *Greater Good Magazine.* https://greatergood.berkeley.edu/article/item/hands_on_research

LaRochelle, J. M., & Karpinski, A. C. (2016). Racial differences in communication apprehension and interprofessional socialization in fourth-year Doctor of Pharmacy students. *American Journal of Pharmaceutical Education, 80*(1), article 8. www.ncbi.nlm.nih.gov/pmc/articles/PMC4776301/pdf/ajpe8018.pdf

Mastrorosa, E. (2019, May 3). Physical contact in different cultures. Blog post. Frontier: Into the wild: The award-winning blog from Frontier. https://frontier.ac.uk/blog/2018/05/03/physical-contact-in-different-cultures

Prochaska, J. O., & DiClemente, C. C. (1983). Stages and processes of self-change of smoking: Toward an integrative model of change. *Journal of Consulting and Clinical Psychology, 51*(3), 390–395. http://dx.doi.org/10.1037/0022-006X.51.3.390

Prochaska, J. O., DiClemente, C. C., & Norcross, J. C. (1992). In search of how people change: Applications to addictive behaviors. *American Psychologist, 47*, 1102–1114. https://doi.org/10.1037/0003-066x.47.9.1102

Provasi, L. (2012, April 4). Physical contact varies by culture. Blog post. Cultural connections: Exploring a world full of diverse cultures and people. https://lizprovasi. wordpress.com/2012/04/04/physical-contact-varies-by-culture/

Rollnick, S., Miller, W. R., & Butler, C. (2008). *Motivational interviewing in health care: Helping patients change behavior.* New York: The Guilford Press.

Sorokowska, A., Sorokowski, P., Hilpert, P., Cantarero, K., Frackowiak, T., Ahmadi, K., … Pierce, J. D., Jr (2017). Preferred interpersonal distances: A global comparison. *Journal of Cross-Cultural Psychology, 48*(4), 577–592. https://doi.org/10.1177/0022022117698039

Suvilehto, J. T., Nummenmaa, L., Harada, T., Dunbar, R. I. M., Hari, R., Turner, R. D., … Ryo, K. (2019). Cross-cultural similarity in relationship-specific social touching. *Proceedings of the Royal Society B: Biological Sciences, 286*(1901). http://doi.org/10.1098/rspb.2019.0467

7

TEAMWORK AND COLLABORATION

Health and social care teams

Human magnificence is beheld in the work of effective interprofessional health and social care teams. Lives are saved, health is promoted, families are strengthened, and communities are uplifted as caring health professionals join their minds, hands, and hearts to offer coordinated responses to problems that one dedicated practitioner alone cannot solve. Immense satisfaction is experienced when health and social care teams composed of diverse members work together and triumph over disease, injury, and despair.

A well-functioning team has many intricacies and nuances. Team members understand and value each other's roles, responsibilities, and contributions. Both inherent and designated leaders are able to think well about the whole and the voices of all team members are elevated. Comradery and collaboration are strong within and across racial and cultural lines, and clients, families, and populations are at the centre and heart of care. Conflict, mistakes, and group dynamics are handled well, and team communication is successful and enhanced through the struggles. How is this ideal team orchestrated, achieved, and replicated?

TeamSTEPPS

Because the establishment of well-functioning teams is both difficult to achieve and also imperative for optimal delivery of health care, increasing efforts are being placed on building stronger teams. Breakdowns in team communication account for many errors in health care. A recent report shows that in the United States, nearly 2,000 patient deaths – and $1.7 billion in malpractice costs – could have been avoided if health care teams had communicated more effectively (Kern, 2016). The most common provider-to-provider communication errors included miscommunication about the patient's condition, poor documentation, and failure to read the medical records. The most common provider-to-patient issues involved inadequately informed consent, an unsympathetic response to a patient's complaint, inadequate education, incomplete follow-up instructions, no information or wrong information given to the patient, and miscommunication due to language barriers (White, 2016).

In response to public outcry against the number of lives lost due to medical errors, the Department of Defense (DoD) and the Agency for Healthcare Research and Quality (AHRQ) in the United States collaboratively developed Team Strategies and Tools to Enhance Performance and Patient Safety (AHRQ, 2020; King et al., 2008), an evidence-based set of tools for improving communication, leadership, and teamwork skills for health care teams that is currently used in health care systems across the globe.

Clear and concise communication

As a basis for clear communication, TeamSTEPPS emphasizes health practitioners placing their full attention on situation monitoring – noticing the status of the patient, team, environment, and progress towards goals. Using the SBAR (Situation – Background – Assessment – Recommendation) technique, health and social care professionals report on critical information that requires immediate attention in a clear and concise manner. In vignette 7.1, Beatrice uses SBAR to ensure that key information is clearly and efficiently shared with her patient's PA after completing her initial PT evaluation. Although SBAR may seem formulaic to a new practitioner, over time, it becomes second nature to communicate using this effective technique.

VIGNETTE 7.1 CLEAR AND CONCISE COMMUNICATION USING SBAR

Beatrice, a PT, shares one-way information with Charlie, a PA.

Situation: Hi Charlie. I'm Beatrice, the physical therapist seeing Mrs Friedman. I noticed her blood pressure (BP) was up; she claimed to feel nauseated.

Background or context: According to my chart review this morning, it didn't look as though high BP was reported.

Assessment: I am wondering if the new medication she began yesterday had an effect today?

Recommendations or requests: Before any physical activity is completed, I recommend she is further assessed for safety.

Assertiveness

In an analysis of 84 root cause analysis reports, Rabøl et al. (2011) found that hesitancy to speak up when concerned about patient safety accounted for 23% of communication errors across six Danish hospitals. Assertiveness has been identified for decades as crucial to effective nursing care (Taylor et al., 2005). Several programmes designed to help nurses speak up have demonstrated how to make positive inroads in this critical area (Omura et al., 2017; Omura et al., 2019; Taylor et al., 2005). Notably, the effective work of Omura et al. (2019) addressed the importance of designing culturally appropriate assertiveness programmes, by taking into account cultural barriers to assertiveness among Japanese nursing students.

Gribble et al. (2018) conducted a longitudinal study and found by the end of their educational programme that Australian undergraduate occupational therapy students reported significant increases in many domains of emotional intelligence (self-perception, decision-making, self-perception, self-actualization, emotional self-awareness, independence, and reality testing), yet scores on assertiveness, problem-solving, and stress tolerance remained relatively low. Similarly, Erbay (2013) found that assertiveness skills in social work students did not improve across a 4-year undergraduate curriculum in Turkey, but remained at a medium level for most students. Male social work students were more assertive than female students, and a significant relationship between the mother's educational level (most mothers' education was at the elementary school level) and assertiveness was noted.

Specific assertiveness techniques

When team members' viewpoints differ from the key leader or decision-maker on a team, TeamSTEPPS suggests several potential assertive responses on behalf of the patient or client that can be offered in a firm and respectful manner: DESC (Describe the Situation with Specific Data – Express Feelings – Suggest Alternatives – Consequences are Shared); and CUS (I'm Concerned – I Feel Uncomfortable – There is a Safety Issue) are excellent assertiveness techniques that are highlighted in vignettes 7.2 and 7.3. The Two Challenge Rule, illustrated in vignette 7.4, recognizes that there are times when an initial assertive statement is ignored. The Two Challenge Rule supports teams in agreeing to the following steps:

- Assertively voice concerns at least two times to ensure your voice has been heard.
- If you are challenged by a team member, you must acknowledge that their concern has been heard.
- If the safety issue still hasn't been addressed, you are asked to take a stronger course of action – possibly utilizing a supervisor or chain of command.

VIGNETTE 7.2 ASSERTIVENESS USING DESC

A social work student, Tara, asserts herself with a physician, Dr Marib, regarding communication in a team meeting.

D – Describe the Situation: *"Hello Dr Marib. I appreciate how well you think about each of your patients. In our team meeting today, I noticed everyone was asked to share updates on their patients except me."*

E – Express: *"I felt too intimidated to speak up in the meeting as a student."*

S – Suggest Alternatives: *"Even though I am a student, I would appreciate it if you would ask me to report in meetings as I have important information to share."*

C – Consequences: *"I know your highest priority is patient care, and they will get better care if all voices at the table are heard."*

VIGNETTE 7.3 RAISING A SAFETY CONCERN BY CUSING

Shelby, an experienced CNA, and John, a student OT, are placing a Thoracic Lumbar Sacral Orthosis (TLSO) brace on a client with a spinal cord injury. Shelby, the CNA states:

C – I am Concerned: *"Hold on, wait for a second, I am concerned."*

U – I am Uncomfortable: *"I am uncomfortable because the brace isn't aligned properly.*

S – This is a Safety Issue: *"If the brace is not aligned with the spine it could be a safety issue and cause permanent damage."*

VIGNETTE 7.4 TWO CHALLENGE RULE

During a discharge meeting with the unit's health care team, Mark, the physician, "made the call" for Michelle, a patient with a right cerebral vascular accident (CVA) to go home. Sarah, the OT, challenged this decision by stating that the patient needed another week at the inpatient facility to further improve instrumental activities of daily living (IADLs). When Mark replied that the client was medically ready to be discharged, the OT stated that although progress had been made, she was not comfortable discharging the patient at this time. The client's goal was to return home and safely complete family meals. Sarah then advocated for the client to continue OT services until this goal had been met, and Mark agreed.

Listening as a conflict resolution tool

While TeamSTEPPS offers many excellent strategies to elevate the voices of team members who might lack the confidence to speak up, the National Coalition Building Institute (NCBI) offers a conflict resolution approach that emphasizes listening. The NCBI Prejudice Reduction Model assumes that no one treats others in a hurtful or disrespectful manner unless they themselves have also been mistreated or disrespected. NCBI participants are trained to separate people from their offending behaviours and to seek attitude change by listening for the place of hurt so that healing can occur. After people have felt validated and listened to regarding their own painful experiences, they are often more open to hearing feedback or information about their offending or prejudicial behaviours and to making significant changes towards behaving differently (Brown & Mazza, 2005). Sandra illustrates these skills in vignette 7.5.

VIGNETTE 7.5 VALIDATE – LISTEN – INFORM

Sandra, the PT, overhears the resident on the treatment team calling their next patient, "The fat one in room 212".

Validate

PT: "You know Dr Smith, I appreciate just how much you care for your patients and give this job your all."

Listen

PT: "Tell me what is up? Why are you calling our next patient 'the fat one'?"
MD: "She is really a large woman and really fat."
PT: "I know you care about her, so why not just call her by her name?"
MD: "I guess what you're saying is I shouldn't be calling her fat?"

Inform

PT: "It is actually very hurtful to most large people to be called 'fat'. In fact, the oppression of large people is called 'fat oppression', and I know the last thing you would want is to be hurtful to your patients."
MD: "You are so right. Thanks for letting me know."

In using the NCBI model, listening is not only at the heart of attitude change but is also at the heart of conflict resolution. When individuals or different groups experience active conflict and disagreement, members on each side are coached in listening to and understanding each other's perspectives. Not surprisingly, those in conflict tend to have great difficulty reporting back the perspective of those in an adversarial role, but can do so with coaching and feedback. As people learn to take turns listening to each other and skilfully inquiring about painful experiences that underlie deeply entrenched attitudes, our common humanity and the potential for conflict resolution emerge.

Appreciation

VIGNETTE 7.6 APPRECIATING ESSENTIAL WORKERS

As someone who was raised working class, Janine, OT, always felt deeply apprecia-tive of the important and unacknowledged work of the CNAs, housekeeping staff,

> *cafeteria workers, staff at the front desk, and transport workers in the hospital. She found it to be a high point in her day when she was able to connect with and appreciate them as frontline workers. Janine found that CNAs, because they spent the most time with patients, always had critical insights on the overall health status and capabilities of her patients.*

The field of Appreciative Inquiry (AI) emphasizes learning from moments of excellence rather than moments of failure (Mohr & Watkins, n.d.). Studies have shown that "organizations grow in the direction of what they repeatedly ask questions about and focus their attention on" (Mohr & Watkins, n.d., p. 2). In other words, the more that people and organizations focus on strengths and achievements rather than shortcomings and problems, the more they tend to flourish. The O.C. Tanner Institute surveyed more than 1,000 employees across the United States and asked, "What is the most important thing your manager or company does (or could do) to cause you to produce great work?" They found that 37% of all respondents and 41% of respondents between 25 and 35 years old identified *recognition* as the most important thing their manager or company could offer to help them produce great work (Sturt et al., 2017). Furthermore, O.C. Tanner's global surveys showed that no matter where you are in the world, appreciation increases employee engagement and innovation. Their inquiries into health care showed that effective recognition of health care workers increased patient satisfaction and clinical outcomes. The role of appreciation in health and social care is further explored in interviews with practitioners in Chapter 11 and in Chapter 12 as a leadership tool.

Giving constructive feedback

Although appreciation and recognition of positive attributes and contributions are extremely important for team functioning, greatness is also achieved through giving and receiving constructive feedback. Every situation is unique, so there is no formula for providing appreciation or constructive feedback. Nonetheless, TeamSTEPPS offers helpful guidelines for the delivery of constructive feedback that encompasses respect and consideration for all individuals concerned.

VIGNETTE 7.7 THE RIPPLE EFFECT OF CONSTRUCTIVE FEEDBACK

Cathy, an OT, was treating an orthopaedic client when Stephan, the PA on the orthopaedic team, walked in to do an evening check before leaving work. He acted as if Cathy were not in the room. He did not acknowledge her or ask if he could interrupt her session. Cathy felt invalidated and undermined in the patient's eyes. The next day she saw Stephan in the documentation room, and since they were the only two there, she brought up her concerns. When Stephan denied her observations and concerns, Cathy informed him that this was not the first time this had occurred, and he might not be aware of his actions. She stated that it was late in the day when the event occurred, and she acknowledged that since it was late in the day, they were both eager to go home. She reiterated that she did not think he had done this intentionally. Cathy also told him she liked him and knew he only had good intentions for his patients. Although that was the end of their conversation, thereafter, Stephan addressed Cathy by her name in the hallway, patient rooms, and asked before interrupting sessions. The physician with whom Stephan worked, who had previously been dismissive to Cathy, also began saying hello and made eye contact with her.

As is beautifully illustrated by Cathy in vignette 7.7, constructive feedback should be:

* timely
* respectful
* specific – relates to a specific task or behaviour that requires correction or improvement
* directed towards improvement
* considerate.

In recognition of the workplace and group dynamics that make it difficult for nurses and other health care practitioners to provide constructive feedback, particularly about uncivil behaviour, Clark (2015), a nurse consultant, offers the following framework (Table 7.1) for providing constructive feedback in challenging conversations:

TABLE 7.1 Clark's Framework for Constructive Feedback

Reflecting, probing, and committing
First ask yourself, "What will happen if I engage in this conversation, and what will happen if I don't?" "What will happen to the patient if I stay silent?" If you decide to engage in a challenging conversation, plan wisely by creating an emotionally and physically safe zone where both parties will be away from others and free of interruptions. Invite a neutral third party if there are power differentials. Use mental rehearsal in preparation for what you will say. Set ground rules together such as one person speaks at a time, maintaining respect, and sticking to objective information. Seek common ground through engaged listening. Make a plan for the follow-up to assess the resolution.

Integration of TeamSTEPPS strategies, such as DESC, as well as other assertive and conflict resolution strategies within Clark's framework can create important inroads towards a more civil and collaborative work environment in health care.

Receiving constructive feedback

VIGNETTE 7.8 THANKS FOR THE FEEDBACK

Jaclyn, an OT, was questioned by Roseanne, her PT colleague, as to why Jaclyn hadn't yet done a cognitive evaluation on her client in the ICU who was delirious. Roseanne had an abrasive style that was offensive to many therapists. Instead of feeling offended, Jaclyn listened to Roseanne's rationale for why the evaluation should be completed as soon as possible, and then explained that when a client was delirious, she preferred to wait 48 hours for the delirium to clear before assessing cognition. Jaclyn appreciated Roseanne for challenging her to stretch her thinking to ensure that the best care possible is offered to their clients.

In their groundbreaking book, *Thanks for the Feedback: The Science and Art of Receiving Feedback Well*, Douglass Stone and Sheila Heen (2014) emphasize developing the art of receiving feedback as a fast track towards personal and professional growth. They expose the key tension around receiving feedback as the pull between:

1. on the one hand, wanting to grow and change
2. on the other hand, wanting to be accepted and loved.

Common triggers that make it difficult to receive constructive feedback include: questioning the truthfulness of the feedback, the complexity of the relationship between the givers and receivers of feedback, and existential identity threats felt in relation to constructive feedback. Strategies for managing these triggers include:

*   developing awareness of our personal triggers and their roots within our own life story
*   cultivating the ability to listen to feedback without being overwhelmed by our feelings
*   learning to say no to some feedback
*   reaching for what is real and true in feedback provided.

Jaclyn, in vignette 7.8, demonstrates the ability to listen to feedback without becoming defensive and to consider what is real in the feedback. The challenge to solicit constructive feedback rather than wait for it to be delivered is an additional step towards being empowered in the feedback process.

Mutual support and recovery from making mistakes

Even with the strong implementation of TeamSTEPPS and other team-building approaches, health care practitioners still make mistakes (see Table 7.2 "Common mistakes made by health and social care practitioners"). With practice, practitioners tend to make fewer mistakes, yet even the most seasoned health care provider still occasionally makes mistakes. Recognizing that one has made a mistake can feel devastating and recovery can feel insurmountable – particularly with mistakes that cause death or serious injury. Due to the severe emotional toll of making serious medical errors, physicians and other health practitioners are increasingly being recognized as the "second victim" in regard to medical errors. Plews-Ogan et al. (2016) used a "post-traumatic growth" model in interviews with 61 physicians who had made a serious medical error. On average, 8 years had passed since the error. Themes reflecting what helped the physician cope and wisdom gained included:

- talking about it – this helped the most, particularly with colleagues who didn't minimize the seriousness of the mistake or dismiss accompanying emotions
- disclosure of the mistake to the patient/family and offering an apology
- forgiving oneself
- having a moral context to help frame doing the right thing
- accepting imperfections and realizing that good doctors make mistakes
- learning and becoming an expert in the area or skill underlying the mistake
- preventing recurrences by improvement in teamwork
- helping others to prevent the same error by teaching

All health practitioners can benefit from the wisdom gained from physicians who have reflected upon their serious mistakes. Since "to err is human", building a cadre of trusted allies who can listen, love, and lift spirits in our hardest moments is an essential dimension of every health practitioner's job.

Further prevention of mistakes: Health literacy and culturally/ linguistically appropriate care

VIGNETTE 7.9 HEALTH LITERACY AND TEACH-BACK

Carl, the PT, was teaching his patient John precautions to take while recovering from a total hip replacement. After demonstrating several important hip precautions, Carl stated, "I know we covered a lot of stuff today, can you remind me of what is the first thing you are supposed to do when you get out of bed? You tell me and I will write it on the whiteboard so you can easily remember?"

TABLE 7.2 Common mistakes made by health and social care practitioners

Physicians (Michon, 2019)	New nurses (NurseJournal.org, 2019)	Social workers (Fanning, 2017)	New occupational therapists (Gribble et al., 2018)	Physical therapists (Dailge, 2012)
Misdiagnosis or delayed diagnosis	Errors with medications	Working harder than the client	Client falls	Going right to the site of pain
Childbirth injuries	Infection control issues	Boundaries	Communication errors that affect the client or colleagues	Not educating patients on the "why" …
Medication errors	Charting and documentation	Underestimating the value of listening and validating	Allowing unsafe client activity	Not listening to the patient sitting right in front of you
Anaesthesia errors	Calling for help without information on hand	Not seeking supervision	Not taking appropriate cautions to protect self	Content with being good, not great
Surgery errors	Falling accidents		Manual handling errors that could harm the therapist or colleagues	Not questioning a possible misdiagnosis or making one's own diagnosis
			Car accidents that could affect patient or therapist	Not marketing and building relationships with other health providers
			Failure to complete paperwork	Utilization of modalities as time killers

With the client, patient, and family at the centre of health and social care teams, using plain language also reduces medical errors and has a profound impact on health outcomes. Raynor (2012) noted that one-third to one-half of people in developed countries have difficulty reading and understanding health information and this has significant, negative consequences on health and mortality. The terms health literacy, health competence, or health ability are used to refer to a client's ability to read and understand health information and to engage in the health care process. Important efforts to enhance health literacy include using plain oral and written language, designing clear written materials, confirming client/patient understanding by having professionals ask the client/patient to repeat what was communicated (teach-back), simplifying overly complex health systems, and implementing programmes to support health professionals in developing their communication skills (Raynor, 2012). Carl, the PT in vignette 7.9 demonstrates effective teach-back by reaching for mutual understanding of what has been shared, and ensuring that his patient is not feeling "quizzed". Key information is reinforced with a visual reminder.

VIGNETTE 7.10 IMPECCABLE ALIGNMENT

Muhammed, the interpreter, stood to the right of Terrance the social worker while they assisted their client Leyla. Muhammed was so skilled in aligning with both Leyla and Terrance that all Leyla's concerns were captured and understood. Muhammed effectively conveyed both of their verbal and non-verbal expressions.

VIGNETTE 7.11 BEYOND WORDS: SALUAREUN KECAP

Rosie, the hospice social worker, connected with Alia, a Sudanese client, by making lots of eye contact as the interpreter shared responses to Rosie's questions about her life story. When Rosie asked what would be helpful to know about Alia to support her in her end of life journey, Alia started talking about her children and how nine of them had been killed in the war, not too long ago. When the interpreter left the room to interact with other family members, Alia started sobbing with Rosie about the loss of her children. Although neither understood a word the other was saying, Rosie and Alia connected deeply. Alia had a cathartic cry that didn't need words.

Understanding the challenges inherent in communicating health information within specific racial and cultural groups only begins to shed light on the challenges in communicating health information across cultural and linguistic differences. The provision of culturally and linguistically appropriate services is an additional complexity that must be addressed to provide optimal care. This is demonstrated in vignette 7.10 where Muhammed uses highly skilled interpretation to assist Terrance in providing excellent care to Leyla, and in vignette 7.11 where Rosie and Alia's connection transcends language barriers. Given the ever-growing diversity in the United States, the HHS Office of Minority Health has released enhanced National Standards for Culturally and Linguistically Appropriate Services (CLAS) in Health and Health Care to help organizations to improve health outcomes for diverse populations (Koh et al., 2014). Google Translate offers an invaluable resource that aids innumerable people in communication across racial and cultural lines.

Standards regarding communication and language assistance include:

- Offer language assistance to individuals who have limited English proficiency or other communication needs, at no cost to them, to facilitate timely access to all health care and services.
- Inform all individuals of the availability of language assistance services clearly and in their preferred language, orally, and in writing.
- Ensure the competence of individuals providing language assistance, recognizing the use of untrained individuals or minors as interpreters should be avoided.
- Provide easy-to-understand print and multimedia materials and signage in the languages commonly used by the populations in the service area.

Koh et al., 2014, p. 199

Implementation of CLAS standards ensures a higher probability of positive health outcomes for racial and ethnic minority groups by fostering the understanding of health information and the engagement in the health process. Evidence also shows that TeamSTEPPS reduces medical errors across diverse populations (Wasserman et al., 2014).

Interprofessional education

In the *Framework for Action on Interprofessional Education & Collaborative Practice* (World Health Organization [WHO], 2010), WHO beautifully captures the potential of interprofessional education (IPE) to promote better health across the globe by fostering strong collaborative practice among health care students. Similar documents, each with their own important nuances, the Canadian Interprofessional Health Collaborative Framework (CIHCF, 2010), and the Core Competencies for Interprofessional Collaborative Practice developed by the Interprofessional Education Collaborative (IPEC, 2016) in the United States, identify similar competency domains in interprofessional education (see Table 7.3). Each approach places the patient, family, caregivers, and populations at the centre of team efforts, and emphasizes team-building skills, understanding and valuing the roles and responsibilities of each health professional, and the development of strong, interprofessional communication skills. Notably, the United

TABLE 7.3 Comparison of interprofessional education competencies

Framework for Action on Interprofessional Education & Collaborative Practice (WHO, 2010)	Canadian Interprofessional Health Collaborative Framework (CIHCF, 2010)	Core Competencies for Interprofessional Collaborative Practice (IPEC, 2016)
Teamwork	Team functioning	Teams and teamwork
	Collaborative leadership	
Role and responsibilities	Role clarification	Roles and responsibilities
Communication	Interprofessional communication and conflict resolution	Interprofessional communication
Ethical practice	(Embedded in other domains)	Values and ethics
Relationship and collaboration with the patient, family, carers, and community as partners	Patient/client/family/ community-centred care	(Embedded in other domains)
Learning and critical reflection		

States updated their IPE document in 2016 and included specific subdomains under roles and responsibilities (RR) and values and ethics (VE) to address cultural effectiveness:

> RR3. Engage diverse professionals who complement one's own professional expertise, as well as associated resources, to develop strategies to meet specific health and healthcare needs of patients and populations.
>
> VE3. Embrace the cultural diversity and individual differences that characterize patients, populations, and the health team.
>
> VE4. Respect the unique cultures, values, roles/responsibilities, and expertise of other health professions and the impact these factors can have on health outcomes.
>
> *IPEC, 2016, pp. 11–12*

Herath et al. (2017) identify interprofessional education as a key factor in addressing not only increasing health needs but also rising costs and shortages in the health care-related workforce globally. They conducted a systematic review to compare IPE and Interprofessional Collaborative Practice (IPCP) across the globe and found that compared with low-resourced (developing) nations, high-resourced (developed) nations had rapid development of IPE programmes and initiatives. In the areas of greatest need, Africa, Latin American, and Caribbean regions, there were few studies addressing IPE. Most IPE programmes reviewed occurred in universities at the undergraduate and/or graduate level and IPE placements occurred

TABLE 7.4 Teamwork and collaboration

Listening and beyond: Dimensions of engaged listening	*Questions for dialogue and connection* Each speaker decides on which question(s) they would like to answer	*Journal/discussion prompts*
Communicating across racial and cultural differences	Talk about building relationships, communicating, and being on teams with people from different racial and cultural groups. What has been challenging?	1. Discuss what you can do to ensure that team members across racial and cultural lines, including yourself, each get a turn to share their perspective.
Interpreters: racial and cultural brokers	• Share any experiences you have had communicating with people who do not speak your first language.	2. Discuss experiences using interpreters and cultural brokers and what you know about racial and cultural literacy.
Health literacy	• Talk about experiences with learning a new language.	3. Discuss the goals you might have regarding learning new languages.
Clear and concise Asserting oneself	• Talk about your strengths and areas for improvement in delivering clear and concise information.	4. Discuss any goals you might have regarding assertive, clear, and concise communication.
Giving and receiving feedback	• Discuss situations in which your communication style is passive, passive-aggressive, assertive, or aggressive, and why?	5. What would help you welcome constructive feedback?
Conflict resolution	• Share positive and negative experiences with receiving feedback.	6. Discuss whether you have been videotaped interacting with others, and whether or not you are ready to implement this tool to improve your communication skills.
Roles and responsibilities	• What strategies can you employ to solicit constructive feedback?	7. Who can you turn to for support when you encounter a communication challenge?
Appreciation (15 + minutes each way)	• Describe any communication challenges you have faced relating to aggression, power dilemmas, resistance, avoidance, etc. What did you do that was effective and what would you do differently in the future?	8. What has it been like to offer support to a peer around communication challenges?
	• Discuss the influence of culture or race in communication challenges you have experienced.	9. Discuss a conflict you did not handle well and identify how you might handle it differently now.
	• What is challenging for you in situations of conflict? How would you like to handle conflict differently? Discuss the influence of culture and race, and if they are factors in how you handle conflict.	10. Discuss the potential role of taking turns at listening to resolve conflict.
	• How was conflict handled in your family as you were growing up?	11. What is it like to appreciate yourself and others?
	• Talk about times when you successfully handled conflict.	
	• Share appreciations of yourself and your listening partner.	

Adapted from: Froehlich, J. (2017), p 110.

in hospitals, communities, or a combination of the two. In each case, target areas were the improvement of knowledge, skills, and attitudes.

Although IPE has many champions across the globe and the support of many qualitative studies, few empirical studies show the effectiveness of IPE efforts. Guraya and Barr (2018) systematically reviewed 8,453 IPE studies and from this database, identified 12 studies that used a pre- and post-intervention design to measure changes in knowledge, attitudes, and skills after an IPE intervention. Although more studies are needed, a meta-analysis of these 12 studies showed statistically significant effectiveness and positive impact of IPE intervention across various disciplines of health care.

Racially and culturally diverse teams

Both TeamSTEPPS and IPE initiatives have made significant contributions towards improving communication and collaborative teamwork within racially and culturally diverse teams. Nonetheless, racial and cultural divisions persist as barriers to optimal team functioning, optimal health care, and optimal health outcomes. Every form of oppression (sexism, homophobia, ageism, classism, anti-Semitism, ableism, etc.) and particularly racism continue to be embedded in all societal institutions, including health care and social care. The reader will become a stronger interprofessional communicator and team player on teams with individuals from diverse backgrounds by engaging in listening partnerships and responding to journal prompts identified in Table 7.4. In Part III, the transformation of racial and cultural lines by deepening connections and activating transformative leadership will be made explicit.

References

Agency for Healthcare Research and Quality (2020, January). *Pocket guide: TeamSTEPPS.* www.ahrq.gov/teamstepps/instructor/essentials/pocketguide.html

Brown, C. R., & Mazza, G. J. (2005). *Leading diverse communities: A how to guide from healing to action* (Revised ed.). San Francisco, CA: Jossey-Bass.

Canadian Interprofessional Health Collaborative (2010). *National interprofessional competency framework.* www.cihc.ca/files/CIHC_IPCompetencies_Feb1210.pdf

Clark, C. M. (2015, November). Conversations to inspire and promote a more civil workplace: Let's end the silence that surrounds incivility. *American Nurse Today, 10*(11), 18–23. www.americannursetoday.com/wp-content/uploads/2015/11/ant11-CE-Civility-1023.pdf

Dailge, R. (2012, February 15). Top 11 mistakes physical therapists make. Blog post. Summit: Professional Education – Instructor Blogs. https://blog.summit-education.com/instructor-blog/the-top-11-mistakes-physical-therapists-make/

Erbay, E. (2013). Assertiveness skills of social work students: A case of Turkey. *Academic Research International, 4*(2), 316–323. www.researchgate.net/publication/285770504_ASSERTIVENESS_SKILL_OF_SOCIAL_WORK_STUDENTS_A_CASE_OF_TURKEY

Fanning, J. (2017, July 28). 4 common social worker mistakes. MSWOnlinePrograms.org. https://mswonlineprograms.org/2017/4-common-social-worker-mistakes/

Froehlich, J. (2017). Effective communication. In K. Jacobs, & N. MacRae (Eds), *Occupational therapy essentials for clinical competence* (3rd ed., pp. 99–132).

Gribble, N., Ladyshewsky, R. K., & Parsons, R. (2018). Changes in the emotional intelligence of occupational therapy students during practice education: A longitudinal study. *British Journal of Occupational Therapy*, *81*(7), 413–422. https://doi.org/10.1177/0308022618763501

Guraya, S. Y., & Barr, H. (2018). The effectiveness of interprofessional education in healthcare: A systematic review and meta-analysis. *Kaohsiung Journal of Medical Sciences*, *34*(3), 160–165. https://doi.org/10.1016/j.kjms.2017.12.009

Herath, C., Zhou, Y., Gan, Y., Nakandawire, N., Gong, Y., & Zuxun, L. (2017, September 26). A comparative study of interprofessional education in global health care: A systematic review. *Medicine (Baltimore)*, *96*(38), e733. https://doi.org/10.1097/md.0000000000007336

Interprofessional Education Collaborative (2016). *Core competencies for interprofessional collaborative practice: Report of an expert panel*. Washington, DC: IPEC. https://hsc.unm.edu/ipe/resources/ipec-2016-core-competencies.pdf

Kern, C. (2016, February 11). Healthcare miscommunication costs 2,000 lives and $1.7 billion. Health IT Outcomes, News feature. www.healthitoutcomes.com/doc/healthcare-miscommunication-costs-lives-and-billion-0001

King, H. B., Battles, J., Baker, D. P., Alonso, A., Salas, E., Webster, J., … Salisbury, M. (2008). TeamSTEPPS™: Team strategies and tools to enhance performance and patient safety. In K. Henriksen, J. B. Battles, M. A. Keyes, & M. L. Grady (Eds), *Advances in patient safety: New directions and alternative approaches:* Vol. 3. *Performance and tools*. Rockville, MD: Agency for Healthcare Research and Quality. www.ncbi.nlm.nih.gov/books/NBK43665/

Koh, H. K., Nadine, G. J., & Alvarez, M. E. (2014). Culturally and linguistically appropriate services: Advancing health with CLAS. *The New England Journal of Medicine*, *371*(2), 198–201. https://doi.org/10.1056/nejmp1404321

Michon, K. (2019). Medical malpractice: Common errors by doctors and hospitals. NOLO. www.nolo.com/legal-encyclopedia/medical-malpractice-common-errors-doctors-hospitals-32289.html

Mohr, B., & Watkins, J. M. (n.d.). *The essentials of appreciative inquiry: A roadmap for creating positive futures*. https://gcatd.org/resources/Documents/Special%20Interest%20Groups%20(SIGs)/Consultants/AI%20article.pdf

NurseJournal.org (2019). The 5 most common mistakes made by new nurses. Nurse Journal: Social Community for Nurses World Wide. https://nursejournal.org/articles/the-5-most-common-mistakes-made-by-new-nurses/

Omura, M., Levett-Jones, T., & Stone, T. E. (2019). Design and evaluation of an assertiveness communication training programme for Japanese nursing students. *Journal of Clinical Nursing*, *28*, 1990–1998. https://doi.org/10.1002/nop2.228

Omura, M., Maguire, J., Levett-Jones, T., & Stone, T. E. (2017). The effectiveness of assertiveness communication training programs for healthcare professionals and students: A systematic review. *International Journal of Nursing Studies*, *76*, 120–128. https://doi.org/10.1016/j.ijnurstu.2017.09.001

Plews-Ogan, M., May, N., Owens, J., Ardelt, M., Shapiro, J., & Bell, S. K. (2016). Wisdom in medicine: What helps physicians after a medical error? *Academic Medicine*, *91*(2), 233–241. https://doi.org/10.1097/acm.0000000000000886

Rabøl, L. I., Andersen, M. L., Østergaard, D., Bjørn, B., Lilja, B., & Mogensen, T. (2011). Descriptions of verbal communication errors between staff: An analysis of 84 root cause analysis-reports from Danish hospitals. *British Medical Journal of Quality & Safety, 20*(3), 268–274. https://qualitysafety.bmj.com/content/20/3/268

Raynor, D. K. (2012). Health literacy. *British Medical Journal, 344*, e2188. doi: 10.1136/bmj. e2188

Stone, D., & Heen, S. (2014). *Thanks for the feedback: The art and science of receiving feedback.* London: Penguin Books.

Sturt, D., Nordstom, T., Ames, K., & Beckstrand, G. (2017). *Appreciate: Celebrating people – inspiring greatness.* Salt Lake City, UT: Tanner Institute Publishing.

Taylor, B., Holroyd, B., Edwards, P., Unwin, A., & Rowley, J. (2005). Assertiveness in nursing practice: An action research and reflection project. *Contemporary Nurse, 20*(2), 234. https://doi.org/10.5172/conu.20.2.234

Wasserman, M., Refrew, M. R., Green, A. R., Lopez, L., Tan-McGrory, A., Brach, C., & Beancourt, J. R. (2014, May–June). Identifying and preventing medical errors in patients with limited English proficiency: Key findings and tools from the field. *Journal of Healthcare Quality, 36*(3), 5–16. https://doi.org/10.1111/jhq.12065

White, J. (2016, February 17). How communication problems put patients, hospitals in jeopardy. Healthcare Business & Technology. www.healthcarebusinesstech.com/communication-patient-harm/

World Health Organization (2010). The WHO Framework for Action. *Journal of Interprofessional Care, 24*(5), 475–478. https://doi.org/10.3109/13561820.2010.504134

PART III

Deepening and restoring connections within and across racial and cultural lines

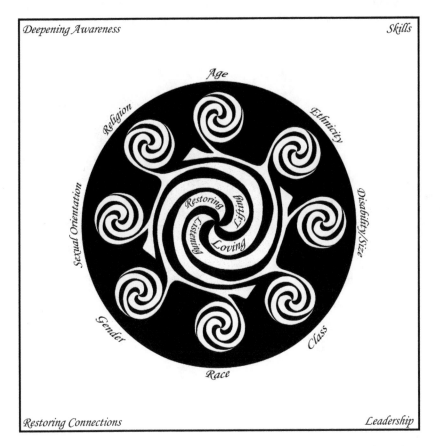

FIGURE 8.1 A model for transforming racial and cultural lines in health and social care

PART III MODEL COMPONENTS
UNDERSTANDING OPPRESSION, INTERNALIZED
OPPRESSION, AND OPPRESSION AND HEALTH
PROCESS: DEEPENING AND RESTORING CONNECTIONS
WITHIN AND ACROSS RACIAL AND CULTURAL LINES

- Gender
- Race
- Class
- Disability/Size
- Ethnicity
- Age
- Religion
- Sexual orientation

8

UNDERSTANDING OPPRESSION AND INTERNALIZED OPPRESSION WITHIN AND ACROSS RACIAL AND CULTURAL IDENTITIES

Historical struggle to survive as humans

Humans are a species indigenous to Africa. For most of our 200,000-year existence as modern humans, homo sapiens lived close to the land as hunter-gatherers. Securing food, water, and finding protection from severe weather, disease, attacking animals, and other humans were ongoing and significant challenges to life. Humans almost became extinct 74,000 years ago due to severe climate (Smithsonian Institution, 2018). Gifted with our genius-size brains, strong upright bodies, opposable thumbs, enormous hearts, the enjoyment of a challenge, a deeply social and occupational nature, and a spirit of cooperation, we were able to forge ahead. We survived extreme conditions by engaging with each other to invent tools, hunt, forage, start fires, and build shelters, and thrived as we developed languages, created food and art, loved deeply, and found merriment in life. We began to migrate out of Africa 120,000 years ago (Tarlach, 2017) and now inhabit every corner of the Earth. Most people on the planet are People of Colour – more accurately described as People of the Global Majority (PGM). As we migrated to different parts of the world, we carried within us a tremendous store of knowledge, ingenuity, capability, gratitude, and love; yet we also brought with us many hurts – grief from untold losses and fears of survival as we journeyed forward.

Beginnings of oppression

In contrast to our existence as hunter-gatherers, the invention of agriculture 12,000 years ago in the Fertile Crescent, an arc-shaped region of the Middle East, enabled humans to produce a surplus of food (National Geographic Partners, 2019). According to Deutsch (2005), one of the founding fathers of the field of conflict resolution, this development had two revolutionary consequences – differentiation of positions within societies and warfare between societies. Some people were freed up from having to produce food, and new occupations emerged including artisans, craftsmen, priests, warriors, and rulers. Social hierarchies, or classism, formed within societies and warfare became a means of further increasing power and domination over groups of people. Humans began to enslave other humans (Deutsch, 2005). Perhaps fuelled by ancient fears for survival and the human tendency to value people in one's own group over others, greed became a dominant force in slave societies. Entitlement, subjugation, and exploitation became organizing forces in slave societies and continued in other oppressive societies. Sumeria is thought to be the birthplace of slavery 11,000 years ago, and it then spread to other parts of the world (Restavek Freedom, 2017). Sexism, the systematic one-way mistreatment of women by men, emerged alongside classism in agricultural societies and placed women as second-class citizens within classist, patriarchal societies (Ananthaswamy & Douglas, 2018).

Evolution of class societies

In Europe and some parts of Asia, slave societies collapsed and were replaced by feudalism. Kings owned all the available land and issued some authority and power to lords and barons over the peasant majority, or serfs (Hirst, 2019). Serfs were essentially peasant farmers who had a few more rights than slaves (Newman, 2019). With the advent of European colonialism or the forceful implantation of their settlements on distant lands, feudalism evolved into various forms of capitalist or owning-class/working-class societies to handle the trade generated from stolen land and resources (Blaut, 1989). While the prospect of economic advantage was the impetus for European colonialism, principles of moral and technological superiority were used to justify the colonization of people in Africa, Asia, and the Americas (Eckhout, 2015).

Europeans accumulated vast amounts of wealth to the detriment and large-scale destruction of Indigenous people they colonized across the globe (Blakemore, 2019). Attempts to destroy or appropriate their languages, cultures, and traditions were only partially successful because of the formidable resistance of people native to the land (Blakemore, 2019; Eckhout, 2015). A vicious and barbaric throw-back to slavery which occurred in the American colonies further fuelled the development of capitalism in America (Blaut, 1989). The large-scale exploitation of African people for their labour was further justified with the invention of racism – the myth of white superiority over Black- and Brown-skinned people (MacKechnie, 2017). Enslavement of African people, combined with the genocide of Native Americans, produced tremendous wealth for the European heritage people who came to be known as white people – people who inhabit the stolen land that is now the centre of global capitalism, the United States (Gilio-Whitaker, 2015; Malik, 2019).

Today, across the globe, an employer or owning class controls most of the wealth and means of producing things that humans depend upon in their daily lives, while workers, both middle- and working-class, are paid a range of wages and salaries in exchange for their labour (Robinson, 2017; Zucchi, 2019). Globally, the combined wealth of the 26 richest people, $1.4 trillion, is as much as the combined wealth of the poorest 3.8 billion, or 50%, of the people on the planet (Oxfam International, 2019). Although capitalism has allowed some groups of people to live longer, and have better health and quality of life, it has wreaked havoc on the lives of many People of the Global Majority (PGM) or Black, Indigenous, and People of Colour (BIPOC) – and continues to do so. For example, in 2018, 10,000 people died every day because they did not have access to health care, while the wealth of billionaires increased by $2.5 billion per day (Oxfam International, 2019).

While humans come from a long lineage of love, caring, creativity, and connection – violence and dominance have also shaped our existence. Vicious exploitation of humans, their land, and their resources has been a key feature in each economic system within hierarchical, oppressive societies and continues to shape the various forms of capitalism today (Lapon, 2011). Modern slavery, forced labour, and subsistence wages continue to exist in capitalist economies throughout the world (Costa, 2015; Restavek Freedom, 2017).

Division and blame as mechanisms of class oppression

Within class societies, multiple forms of oppression (racism, sexism, gay oppression, anti-Semitism, disability oppression, language oppression, etc.) emerged as tools to divide and pit oppressed groups against one another (Nagain, 2018). This tactic has served and still serves to divert the hostility and attention of the oppressed and exploited working class and poor people away from the ruling or owning class in various countries, and instead directs their hostility towards the so-called "problem" or target group (i.e. Jews, immigrants, People of the Global Majority, etc.).

For example, anti-Semitism, the oppression of Jews, is sometimes thought of as the oldest hate. Early Christianity vilified Jews, rather than Roman society, for "killing Christ" (Phillips, 2018). In the Middle Ages, as Jews settled on various lands throughout Europe, scapegoating continued. As literate people, unlike most Christians at the time, Jews were able to acquire the skills necessary to serve as money lenders, tax collectors, and public officials (Botticini & Eckstein, 2013). At some point, the European nobility deliberately excluded Jews from other occupations as a tactical move to position Jews as the visible agent of oppression towards peasants and tenant farmers (Hatfutsot, 2017). When non-Jews organized to resist their oppressive conditions, their hatred, resentment, and violence were directed towards Jews instead of towards the rulers of the lands they inhabited (Jews for Racial & Economic Justice, 2017). The Holocaust, the most extreme and large-scale example of anti-Semitic violence, was fuelled by Nazi propaganda which targeted and blamed Jews for the impoverishment of the German people after World War I. The scapegoating and extreme destruction of Jews and Jewish communities have occurred over and over again throughout history – always blaming Jews for society's problems. Overt anti-Semitism, such as the bombing of synagogues, desecration of Jewish cemeteries, and other acts of violence against Jews, and the more covert examples such as stereotyping of Jews as controlling the media and banking industries, persist today and divert movements for justice and equality (Jews for Racial & Economic Justice, 2017).

Anti-Semitism paved the way for the vicious targeting of other groups. In the United States today as wealth inequality deepens, immigrants of colour are increasingly blamed for myriad social problems – stealing jobs from the white working-class people; increased crime, drug use, assaults against Americans; and preying upon welfare and health care benefits (Rahimi & Boyd, 2019). Only a divided people, misinformed about the nature of oppression and the dynamics of classism, would target each other rather than the ruling elites who control most of the wealth, the means of production, and the political power in societies (Jews for Racial & Economic Justice, 2017). Paradoxically, while our species as a whole has benefitted immensely from advances achieved within class societies in many realms, the core values of exploitation, greed, and profitability within classist systems have caused the loss of countless lives, inflicted misery and suffering among millions of people, damaged the human psyche, and now place human existence and the survival of many plant and animal species on Earth in jeopardy because of the massive destruction of the whole planet.

Oppression operationalized

Oppression, the one-way systematic mistreatment of one group of people by another group of people or by society, involves the unjust, cruel, harsh, and deadly exercise of power and control over various targeted groups in society – it can be both conscious and unconscious (Bell, 2010; Community Tool Box, 2019; Palmer et al., 2019; Ruth, 2006). Humans cannot be oppressed unless tremendous mistreatment, violence, coercion, and invalidations are strategically and systematically placed upon them by those in oppressor roles (Freire, 1993). Oppression is enacted in hierarchical structures that are embedded in every institution within some societies – political, legal, and governmental structures; reproduction and child-rearing, marriage, and family life; educational systems, religion, sports, and entertainment industries; housing; mass media; military and police forces; penal institutions; welfare; pornography and sex industries; health care systems; economy and work; and food industries (Chinook Fund, 2010; Freire, 1993; Kelly & Varghese, 2018; Palmer et al., 2019).

Conditioning of the oppressor: Forces that shape oppressor identity

Oppressor roles are formed through the instalment and reinforcement of prejudice, bias, stereotypes, and misinformation about different groups of people within every institution in society (DiAngelo, 2018; Ruth, 2006). The development of prejudice

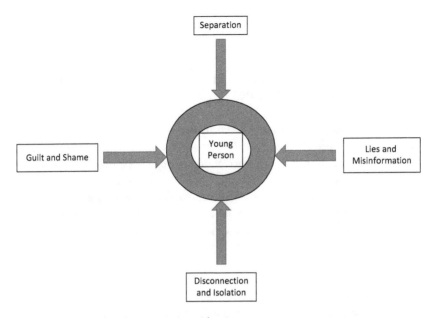

FIGURE 8.2 Forces that shape oppressor identity

and biases and the conditioning to play oppressive roles begins when people are young and continues throughout the life span (DiAngelo, 2018; Dunham et al., 2008; Jackins and others, 2002). The forces which shape oppressor identity are identified in Figure 8.2. Young people in oppressor groups are often separated from people who are targeted by oppression and are taught and told vicious lies and misinformation about those groups. These lies and misinformation become the basis for stereotypes and prejudice towards groups targeted by oppression. This can cause people in oppressor roles to be fearful and hateful towards groups targeted by oppression. Many people in oppressor roles are often disconnected from their inherently loving selves and from other people in the oppressor role. They tend to feel very guilty and ashamed.

While humans have varying consciousness of the prejudice and stereotypes they hold towards different groups, studies on implicit bias reveal that many pre-conceived notions of groups of people other than our own, both favourable and unfavourable, lie within our unconscious psyche (Payne et al., 2018). Awareness of overt acts of discrimination and aggression and smaller acts of everyday aggressive insults lies on a similar continuum (Sue et al., 2018). While some acts of oppression are calculated and strategic, many are conducted on an unaware level due to the very nature of the earlier damage inflicted upon people acting as agents of oppression (Jackins and others, 2002). No human is born with a desire to oppress others – they are systematically conditioned to play oppressive roles by society (Jackins and others, 2002).

Microaggressions

VIGNETTE 8.1 ARROGANCE SPRINKLED WITH A TOUCH OF POLITENESS: ÆɪƏ.GƏNS

Mato, a PA, proudly displayed all of his degrees visibly on the wall behind his desk. He was especially proud of his first – an associate degree from Haskell Indian Nations University. This particular degree was a tribute to his hard work, determination, and perseverance and that of his family and his tribal ancestors. Paul, a white PA, shared an office with Mato. He looked curiously at the degree, and with a tone of arrogance and condescension, asked, "I wonder why I have never heard of that university. Is it very good? Is it accredited? Where does it rank?"

Smaller, everyday oppressive acts of aggression, or microaggressions, are defined by Sue et al. as "derogatory slights or insults directed at a target person or persons who are members of an oppressed group" (2018, p. 25). These scholars identify three forms of microaggression: – microassaults, microinsults, and microinvalidations. Microassaults are overt verbal or non-verbal acts of discrimination that are derogatory towards oppressed groups. For example, the use of racial epithets towards People of the Global Majority or slurs against gay people are considered microassaults. Microassaults differ from assaults because physical harm is not involved. Microinsults are unintentional behaviours or verbal comments that are demeaning, rude, or insensitive towards a person's racial and/or cultural identity. A common example of a microinsult is when a white middle-class person unawarely assumes and conveys that a person of colour or working-class person is of inferior status or lacks intelligence simply because of their racial or class background. In vignette 8.1, Paul unintentionally insults Mato as he inquires about Haskell Indian Nations University. Microinvalidations are also unintentional and are exhibited in comments or behaviours that dismiss the thoughts, feelings, or experiential reality of a targeted group. A common microinvalidation happens when individuals claim that they are colourblind and only see humans as humans. This microinvalidation dismisses the reality that People of Colour experience the stressful impact of living with racism on a daily basis (Sue et al., 2018).

Due to the pervasive nature of implicit bias, the reader is encouraged to explore their own unconscious or automatic biases towards different groups by taking a variety of the implicit association tests developed by Project Implicit (2011) at www.project.implicit.net. Project Implicit is an international collaborative research effort initiated by psychologists at Harvard University, the University of Virginia, and the University of Washington to educate the public on hidden biases, collect data on hidden biases, and translate data to address diversity within organizations.

Internalized oppression

VIGNETTE 8.2 AFRICAN HAIRITAGE – AFRIKEN ERITAJ

Angela, a social worker of African heritage yearned for the connection that only Black women could provide her. Yet she also knew that internalized oppression divided her from other Black women. When Angela was approached by Betty, a white resident in the nursing home where she was employed. Betty expressed concern that Mercy, a CNA of Haitian heritage, was not taking the best care of her. Betty adamantly said, "Mercy has such big, wild, and out of control hair. I don't think she knows what clean is and I don't like her touching my hair". It made Angela's job difficult when white residents complained to her about Mercy's hair though secretly, she harboured similar thoughts: "Why does she wear her hair nappy like that? Doesn't she know that Afros, braids, or dreads have no place in nursing? It looks so unprofessional and gives nursing a bad name." Angela was saddened to remember how residents had also complimented her own hair, sharing their preference for hair that was flowing, shiny, and controlled, and how she did not discourage them from touching her hair.

While oppression is deeply harmful physically, psychologically, spiritually, and emotionally towards target groups, one of the most damaging consequences of oppression is the phenomenon of internalized oppression. Internalized oppression is the internalization of negative messages from the oppressor that are turned in on oneself and one's own group (Community Tool Box, 2019; David, 2015). Hence, explicit and implicit bias is found not only in the conscious and unconscious mind of the oppressor, but also in the conscious and unconscious minds of oppressed groups about themselves and each other (Ashburn-Nardo et al., 2003; Kendi, 2019).

Examples of internalized oppression can be seen within all oppressed groups. Institutionalized and racist experiences of vicious enslavement, violence, mistreatment, exploitation, subjugation, and invalidation of Black people from dominant white society results in enormous self-invalidation among Black people and the pull to invalidate and mistrust other Black people. This is exemplified between Angela and Mercy in vignette 8.2. The oppression of all women has left women believing they are of lesser value and are less capable than men and this fuels the tremendous backstabbing, competition, preoccupation with appearance, and gossiping that women engage in. The oppression of classism leaves the working class seeing themselves as less intelligent and less important than middle- and owning-class people, and they denigrate each other for being stupid and unworthy. For every oppressed group – women, People of the Global Majority, people with disabilities, LGBTQ+ individuals, the working class, religious and cultural groups, colonized people, people who don't speak the majority language, etc. – the struggle not to break under the weight and divisiveness of internalized oppression can seem formidable.

Lateral or horizontal violence in health care

Internalized oppression is a fundamental interlocking factor in maintaining all forms of oppression within a class system which mandates that its participants justify and agree to the subjugation of self and others of their racial and cultural group. This extends to health care professionals who, due to their oppression as workers within a class system, mistreat and denigrate each other with mistreatment and microaggressions. The terms horizontal and lateral violence are used to describe the vicious backstabbing, gossiping, bullying, incivility, and mistreatment that occurs in the workplace towards those with less power or status. Nursing has been identified as the profession most at risk for horizontal violence because their lack of power and control within physician-dominated medical hierarchies obscure the value of nursing (Vessey et al., 2010). Between 46% and 100% of nurses report experiences of lateral violence (Stanley et al., 2007).

> ### VIGNETTE 8.3 FIGHTING LATERAL VIOLENCE TOGETHER
>
> *Carmen, a labour and delivery nurse, confides in Donna, also a nurse and her closest friend at work, that she is burnt out from her job – not because of the work, but because of the constant backstabbing by other nurses who disagree with her more natural approach to the birthing process. Donna agrees with Carmen that lateral violence is the worst part of the nursing profession and assures Carmen she has her back – they will fight this together.*

Griffin (2004) identified examples of outward behavioural manifestations of lateral violence – making faces or raising eyebrows in response to a colleague, making rude or demeaning comments, acting in ways that undermine the ability to help others, sabotaging one another by withholding information, group infighting, scapegoating, passive-aggressive communication, gossiping and failure to respect privacy or breaking confidences. New nursing graduates are particularly vulnerable to experiencing lateral violence, and this results in higher absenteeism, reduced work satisfaction, increased stress, and a desire to leave their job (Falletta, 2017). In 2019, the turnover rate of bedside nursing in the United States was 15.9% and 26.5% for CNAs (Nursing Solutions Incorporated, 2020). Vignette 8.3 is an example of lateral violence and the potential for strong partnerships to break this vicious pattern among nurses.

A common human experience: Playing both oppressor and oppressed roles

Societies condition most, if not all, humans, into playing both oppressor and oppressed roles at different times in our lives. For example, what child has not only been picked on, but has also picked on another child because of age or some other identity? What parent has not acted oppressively towards their child because they did not know what else to do in desperate and isolated moments? Nonetheless, the experience of being in the oppressor role is radically different from being in an oppressed or victim role.

Mutuality: Sharing stories of racial-cultural identities and experiences with oppression

VIGNETTE 8.4 CULTURAL FASHION SHOW

Miranda, a PT, and her peers organized a cultural fashion show at work. It was deeply satisfying to see hierarchies and divisions in the workplace melt as staff across the hospital from all backgrounds shared pride in their beautiful regalia, music, and food in celebrations of their racial and cultural identities. People who generally never talked with each other laughed and delighted in this cultural sharing.

Talking about oppression can be difficult yet also deeply desirable, satisfying, and liberating for both oppressed people and people in oppressor roles. Sharing our rich and varied racial, cultural, and linguistic identities through food, stories, poetry, music, dance, and other creative arts can facilitate a process of mutuality. As we see in vignette 8.4, Miranda is particularly pleased with how her cultural fashion show dissolved some of the divisions within the workplace and facilitated new relationships.

Brooks et al. (2018) conducted a concept analysis of culturally sensitive communication in health care and determined that understanding one's own culture is an essential first step before learning about other cultures. By building awareness and pride and discovering bonds to our own racial and cultural identities first, we can strengthen connections within ourselves and with others and then share difficult and informative experiences of oppression, implicit bias, microaggressions, and internalized oppression. Many listening exchanges may need to occur within racial, cultural, and linguistic identity groups before enough safety is generated to share hurtful experiences related to oppression, microaggressions, and internalized oppression with people in other identity groups.

TABLE 8.1 Partnerships for understanding oppression and internalized oppression within and across racial and cultural lines

Listening to understand racial and cultural identities and experiences with oppression	Questions for dialogue and connection Each speaker decides on which question(s) they would like to answer	Journal/discussion prompts
Oppression and internalized oppression across racial and cultural lines (15 + minutes each way)	• What is your racial, cultural, and ethnic background? • What are you proud of and what are challenges related to your racial, cultural, and ethnic heritage? • Were you ever a member of a racial or cultural minority in your neighbourhood, school, church, or social situation as you were growing up? If so, what was this like? • Were there ever times you felt mistreated as a member of a particular group? What was this like? • Discuss what it has been like to stand against the mistreatment of other racial and cultural groups. • If you live in a country different from that of your ethnic origin, why did you or your ancestors come to the country you are living in now? Discuss if oppression was a factor. • What makes you proud to be a citizen of _____ country and how would you like your country to be different? • Discuss the results of several implicit bias tests with people from your own racial and cultural groups – what did you learn, what surprised you, and what action can you take to reduce your own implicit biases?	1. What conditions enable you to open up about difficult experiences? 2. Discuss if you felt comfortable talking with your listening partner about times when you felt mistreated. 3. Discuss times you made friends with someone from a different racial, cultural, or ethnic group. 4. Discuss times when you have made mistakes in interactions with people from different ethnic, racial, and cultural groups. 5. What holds you back from building relationships across racial, cultural, and ethnic differences? What would help you take risks in building relationships across racial, cultural, and ethnic differences? 6. What is it like to have a dialogue about race, culture, and ethnicity? 7. Discuss a time when someone from a racial or cultural group different from your own pointed out a microaggression or oppressive behaviour you directed at them. How did you feel, how did you respond and share if you were able to learn from this experience? If so, what factors enabled you to learn from this experience?

Adapted from: Froehlich, J. (2017), p 110.

Table 8.1 offers listening partners questions and discussion/journal prompts that guide exploration of oppression and internalized oppression in each others' lives. Subsequent chapters will explore the impact of oppression on health and the complexity of healing from experiences as oppressed people and as oppressors. The transformative power of developing friendships and listening partnerships within and across racial and cultural lines is a foundation for action against oppression that will be highlighted.

References

Ananthaswamy, A., & Douglas, K. (2018, April 18). The origins of sexism: How men came to rule 12,000 years ago. *New Scientist*. www.newscientist.com/article/mg23831740-400-the-origins-of-sexism-how-men-came-to-rule-12000-years-ago/

Ashburn-Nardo, L., Knowles, M. L., & Monteith, M. J. (2003). Black Americans' implicit racial associations and their implications for intergroup judgment. *Social Cognition, 21*(1), 61–87. https://doi.org/10.1521/soco.21.1.61.21192

Bell, L. A. (2010). Theoretical foundations. In M. Adams, W. J. Blumenfeld, R. Castañeda, H. Hackman, M. Peters, & X. Zúñiga (Eds), *Readings for diversity and social justice* (2nd ed., pp. 20–25). New York: Routledge.

Blakemore, E. (2019, February 19). What is colonialism: A history of colonialism is one of brutal subjugation of indigenous peoples. National Geographic: Culture. www.nationalgeographic.com/culture/topics/reference/colonialism/

Blaut, J. (1989). Colonialism and the rise of capitalism. *Science & Society, 53*(3), 260–296. Available at: www.jstor.org/stable/40404472

Botticini, M., & Eckstein, Z. (2013). Were the Jews moneylenders out of necessity? *Reform Judaism*. https://reformjudaismmag.org/past-issues/spring2013/jews-moneylenders

Brooks, L. A., Manias, E., & Bloomer, M. J. (2019). Culturally sensitive communication in healthcare: A concept analysis. *Collegian, 26*(3), 383–391. www.collegianjournal.com/article/S1322-7696(17)30315-3/pdf

Chinook Fund (2010, October). The four "I's" of oppression. www.coloradoinclusivefunders.org/uploads/1/1/5/0/11506731/the_four_is_of_oppression.pdf

Community Tool Box (2019). Chapter 27: Cultural competence in a multicultural world: Section 3: Healing from the effects of internalized oppression. Tools to change our world. https://ctb.ku.edu/en/table-of-contents/culture/cultural-competence/healing-from-interalized-oppression/main

Costa, D. (2015, June 16). The true cost of low prices is exploited workers. Economic Policy Institute. Working Economics blog. www.epi.org/blog/true-cost-of-low-prices-is-exploited-workers/

David, E. J. R. (2015, September 30). Internalized oppression: We need to stop hating ourselves. *Psychology Today*. www.psychologytoday.com/us/blog/unseen-and-unheard/201509/internalized-oppression-we-need-stop-hating-ourselves

Deutsch, M. (2005, March). The nature and origins of oppression. Beyond Intractability. www.beyondintractability.org/essay/nature-origins-oppression

DiAngelo, R. (2018). *White fragility: Why it's so hard for white people to talk about racism.* Boston, MA: Beacon Press.

Dunham, Y., Baron, A. S., & Banaji, M. R. (2008). The development of implicit intergroup cognition. *Trends in Cognitive Sciences, 12*(7), 248–253. https://doi.org/10.1016/j.tics.2008.04.006

Eckhout, A. (2015, April 30). Justification of a nation. Edges of Empire. https://people.smu. edu/knw2399/2015/04/30/the-justification-of-a-nation/

Falletta, E. (2017, September 14). Lateral violence in the workplace. *Johns Hopkins Nursing*. https://magazine.nursing.jhu.edu/2017/09/lateral-violence-workplace/

Freire, P. (1993). *Pedagogy of the oppressed*. Manhattan, NY: Penguin Random House.

Froehlich, J. (2017). Effective communication. In K. Jacobs, & N. MacRae (Eds), *Occupational therapy essentials for clinical competence* (3rd ed., pp. 99–132).

Gilio-Whitaker, D. (2015, February 23). Genocide and slavery: The evil twins of colonialism. Indian Country Today. https://newsmaven.io/indiancountrytoday/archive/ genocide-and-slavery-the-evil-twins-of-colonialism-KerGe7W3iEeUgILWu0ljYg/

Griffin, M. (2004). Teaching cognitive rehearsal as a shield for lateral violence: An intervention for newly licensed nurses. *Journal of Continuing Education in Nursing, 35*(6), 257–262. https://doi.org/10.3928/0022-0124-20041101-07

Hatfutsot, B. (2017, August 24). Jews and money in anti-Semitic views. Museum of the Jewish People at Beit Hatfutsot. https://www.bh.org.il/blog-items/jews-money-anti-semitic-views/

Hirst, K. K. (2019, May 23). Feudalism: A political system of Medieval Europe and elsewhere. ThoughtCo. www.thoughtco.com/feudalism-political-system-of-medieval-europe-170918

Jackins, T. and others (2002). *Working together to end racism: Healing from the damage caused by racism*. Seattle, WA: Rational Island Publishers.

Jews for Racial and Economic Justice (2017, November). *Understanding antisemitism: An offering to our movement*. www.jfrej.org/assets/uploads/JFREJ-Understanding-Antisemitism-November-2017-v1-3-2.pdf

Kelly, D. C., & Varghese, R. (2018). Four contexts of institutional oppression: Examining the experiences of Blacks in education, criminal justice and child welfare. *Journal of Human Behavior in the Social Environment, 28*(7), 874–888. https://doi.org/10.1080/ 10911359.2018.1466751

Kendi, I. X. (2019). *How to be an antiracist*. New York: One World.

Lapon, G. (2011, September 28). What do we mean by exploitation? SocialistWorker.org. https://socialistworker.org/2011/09/28/what-do-we-mean-exploitation

MacKechnie, J. (2017, April 20). Justifying slavery: The changing shape of the slave trade in the medieval Mediterranean. *History Today*. www.historytoday.com/justifying-slavery

Malik, K. (2019, March 16). The history and politics of white identity. Pandaemonium. https://kenanmalik.com/2019/03/16/the-history-and-politics-of-white-identity/

Nagain, R. (2018, January 24). Working-class unity is the key to ending racism and male supremacy. People's World. www.peoplesworld.org/article/working-class-unity-is-key-to-ending-racism-and-male-supremacy/

National Geographic Partners (2019). The development of agriculture: The farming revolution. *National Geographic*. www.nationalgeographic.org/article/development-agriculture/

Newman, S. (2019). Serfs in the Middle Ages. The Finer Times. www.thefinertimes.com/ Middle-Ages/serfs-in-the-middle-ages.html

Nursing Solutions Incorporated (2020). 2020 NSI national healthcare retention & RN staffing report. NSI: A Solutions Group Company. www.nsinursingsolutions.com/ Documents/Library/NSI_National_Health_Care_Retention_Report.pdf

Oxfam International (2019). 5 shocking facts about extreme global inequality and how to even it up. Oxfam International. www.oxfam.org/en/even-it/5-shocking-facts-about-extreme-global-inequality-and-how-even-it-davos

Palmer, G. L., Fernández, J. S., Lee, G., Masud, H., Hilson, S., Tang, C., … Bernai, I. (2019). Oppression and power. In L. A. Jason, O. Glantsman, J. F. O'Brien, & K. N. Ramian (Eds), *Introduction to community psychology: Becoming an agent of change*. Creative Commons Attribution. https://press.rebus.community/introductiontocommunitypsychology/

Payne, K., Niemi, L., & Doris, J. M. (2018, March 27). How to think about "implicit bias". *Scientific American*. www.scientificamerican.com/article/how-to-think-about-implicit-bias/

Phillips, G. (2018). Anti-Semitism: How the origins of history's oldest hatred still hold sway today. The Conversation. https://theconversation.com/antisemitism-how-the-origins-of-historys-oldest-hatred-still-hold-sway-today-87878

Project Implicit (2011). Implicit social cognition. www.projectimplicit.net/

Rahimi, A., & Boyd, J. W. (2019, January 11). Blaming others: What's behind the talk about immigrants. *Psychology Today*. www.psychologytoday.com/us/blog/almost-addicted/201901/blaming-others-what-s-behind-the-talk-about-immigrants

Restavek Freedom (2017). The history of slavery. Restavek Freedom: Ending Child Slavery in Haiti. https://restavekfreedom.org/2018/09/11/the-history-of-slavery/

Robinson, W. I. (2017, August 3). Global capitalism: Reflections on a brave new world. resilience. www.resilience.org/stories/2017-08-03/global-capitalism/

Ruth, S. (2006). *Leadership and liberation*. New York: Routledge.

Smithsonian Institution (2018, September 14). What does it mean to be human? Smithsonian: National Museum of Natural History. http://humanorigins.si.edu/human-characteristics/humans-change-world

Stanley, K., Martin, M., Michel, Y., Welton, M., & Nemeth, S. (2007). Examining lateral violence in the nursing workplace. *Issues in Mental Health Nursing, 28*(11), 1247–1265. https://doi.org/10.1080/01612840701651470

Sue, D. W., Capodilupo, C. M., Nadal, K. L., Rivera, D. P., & Torino, G. C. (2018). *Microaggression theory: Influence and implications*. Hoboken, NJ: John Wiley & Sons.

Tarlach, G. (2017, December 1). It's official: Timeline for human migration gets a rewrite. *Discover: Science for the Curious*. http://blogs.discovermagazine.com/deadthings/2017/12/07/human-migration-rewrite/#.XVCV4ZNKiqA

Vessey, J. A., DeMarco R., & DiFazio R. (2010). Bullying, harassment, and horizontal violence in the nursing workforce: The state of the science. *Annual Review of Nursing Research, 28*, 133–157. https://doi.org/10.1891/0739-6686.28.133

Zucchi, K. (2019, May 7). Main characteristics of capitalist economies. Investopedia. www.investopedia.com/articles/investing/102914/main-characteristics-capitalist-economies.asp

9

OPPRESSION, HEALTH, AND WELLBEING

Consequences of oppression on health and wellbeing

Prior to the coronavirus pandemic, the World Health Organization (WHO) cited notable progress towards its aspirational goal of achieving the highest standard of health for all regardless of race, religion, political belief, economic, or social condition (WHO, 2019a). Since 1950, life expectancy had increased by 25 years across the globe. Six million fewer children died before they reached their fifth birthday in 2016 compared with 1990. Smallpox had been eliminated and polio was close to being eradicated. Measles, malaria, and debilitating tropical diseases as well as mother-to-child transmission of HIV and syphilis had been defeated in many countries (WHO, 2019a). Yet, half the world still lacked access to essential health services (WHO, 2017). Globally, more than 800 million people did not have enough food to eat, yet rates of obesity were on the rise (WHO, 2019b). One in three people did not have adequate access to clean drinking water to sustain health (WHO, 2019c). Thousands died each day from diarrhoea caused by inadequate drinking water, sanitation, and hand hygiene (WHO, 2019d). While the coronavirus pandemic now threatens numerous global health gains, poor nations face catastrophic losses (Malley & Malley, 2020).

The link between poverty, poor health, and shorter lives has been understood for many years. Socioeconomic status (SES), including educational level, occupation, income, and assets are major determinants of health (WHO, 2019e). The wealth–health gradient exposes the reality that every step on the rung towards wealth means increases in longevity and health status (Marmot, 2017). Yet poverty alone does not explain the health disparities between groups of people. For example, while police violence is a leading cause of death for all young men in the United States, Black men and women and American Indian and Alaskan Native men and women are significantly more likely than white men and women to be killed by the police, and Latino men are also more likely to be killed by police than white men (Edwards et al., 2019). Black men are particularly at risk for destruction – they are 2.5 times more likely than white men to be killed by police over the course of their lifetime.

Williams et al. (2019) cite numerous studies that document higher rates of disease and death, earlier onset of illnesses, the more aggressive progression of the disease and poorer survival for Blacks (or African Americans), Native Americans (or American Indians and Alaska Natives), Native Hawaiians and Other Pacific Islanders in the United States – even after adjustment for socioeconomic status (SES). Declining health for Mexican immigrants residing in the United States for more than 20 years was found not to differ from that of African Americans. The tangible and intangible trauma of racism has dire health consequences that are only worsening in the coronavirus pandemic (Mahler et al., 2020; Yancy, 2020).

Social determinants of health

The World Health Organization broadly defines the conditions in which people are born, grow up, live, work, and age as the social determinants of health (SDH) (WHO, 2019e). WHO acknowledges that these conditions are influenced by the unequal distribution of money, power, and resources at the global, national, and local levels and indicts the social determinants of health as mostly responsible for health inequities or the unfair and avoidable differences in health status seen both within and between nations (WHO, 2019e). It has been estimated that SDH contribute 60% to health outcomes, while our healthcare system contributes just 20%, and genetics contributes 20% to health outcomes (Braveman & Gottlieb, 2014).

Healthy People 2020 in the United States also links health disparities to social, economic, and/or environmental disadvantage and identifies five key areas as social determinants of health (see Table 9.1) (Office of Disease Prevention and Health Promotion, 2019a). Healthy People 2020's overarching goal is to achieve health equity, eliminate disparities, and improve the health of all groups. Healthy People 2020 places specific attention on disparities experienced by people based on the racial or ethnic group; religion; socioeconomic status; gender; age; mental health; cognitive, sensory, or physical disability; sexual orientation or gender identity; geographic location; or other characteristics historically linked to discrimination or exclusion (Office of Disease Prevention and Health Promotion, 2019b). Similarly, Canadian Professors of Nursing, McGibbon et al. (2008) include identity groups in their analysis of social determinants of health; they more explicitly argue that *systemic oppression* produces poor health.

Oppressed groups: People under threat

McGibbon (2012) describes oppressed groups as *people under threat*. The everyday experiences of poverty, racism, sexism, homophobia, colonialism, etc. threaten the

TABLE 9.1 Healthy People 2020 social determinants of health

Economic stability	Education
• Employment	• Early childhood education and development
• Food insecurity	• Enrolment in higher education
• Housing instability	• High school graduation
• Poverty	• Language and literacy
Social and community context	**Health and health care**
• Civic participation	• Access to health care
• Discrimination	• Access to primary care
• Incarceration	• Health literacy
• Social cohesion	

Neighborhood and built environment
• Access to foods that support healthy eating patterns
• Crime and violence
• Environmental conditions
• Quality of housing

Source: Office of Disease Prevention and Health Promotion (2019a).

health, wellbeing, and the very existence of oppressed groups. Insecurity related to basic human needs – housing, food, clean water, access to medical care, and safety from violence – generates toxic stress. This daily stress load affects the body's stress managing systems and leads to high blood pressure, type 2 diabetes, obesity, cancer, ulcers, chronic stomach problems, allergies, eczema, autoimmune diseases, health aches, kidney and liver disease, and reduced immunity (Halter & Varcarolis, 2014.) Furthering the insult, the *medicalization of oppression* reframes the mental anguish generated by food insecurity, domestic violence, racial profiling, homophobia, and housing instability as psychiatric conditions that can be labelled and medicated (McGibbon, 2012). Yet no pill eliminates poverty, racism, sexism, or other forms of oppression (McGibbon, 2012).

Health across identity groups

Compelling research on the health consequences of oppression addresses the intersection of multiple oppressions, including the effects of the coronavirus pandemic, on targeted groups. Glaring examples of the damage to health caused by the oppression experienced by diverse groups are highlighted in Appendix D, "Health and wellbeing of people under threat." By reading these examples, you are invited to become increasingly curious, aware, and ready to take courageous action to reduce health disparities experienced across racial and cultural groups.

Unequal societies

To some extent, the more unequal a society is, the greater the experience of "threat" is to *all* members of that society. Epidemiological research shows that high levels of inequality negatively affect the health of even the richest sector of the population (Wilkinson & Pickett, 2009) (see Figure 9.1). Inequality within a society destroys social cohesion which in turn generates high levels of stress, fear, and insecurity for everyone (Pickett & Wilkinson, 2015). When everyone lives under "threat", the health of everyone is damaged.

The United States, the wealthiest nation in the world, and the only high-income country without universal health care is also the most unequal country among wealthy nations (Davis, 2018; McFarland, 2018). Additionally, the United States spends more on health care as a share of the economy, nearly twice as much as the average of other high-income countries, yet has the lowest life expectancy and the highest suicide rate among wealthy nations (Tikkanen & Abrams, 2020). Sadly, Woolf and Schoomaker (2019) found that despite enormous gains in life expectancy between 1959 and 2016, the United States stands out among high-income countries for declining life expectancy in recent years. They found that people of all racial groups in the United States are more likely to die before 65 than people in other wealthy nations – primarily because of what some refer to as "deaths of despair" – drug overdose, alcohol abuse, and suicide. Fatalities related to obesity

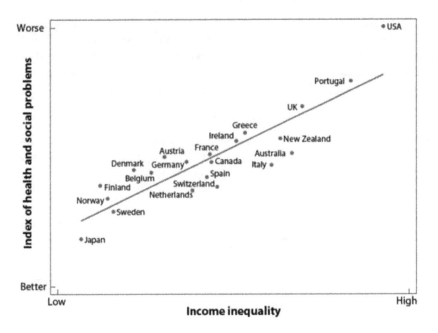

FIGURE 9.1 Index of health and social problems in relation to income inequality in rich countries

and diverse organ diseases are also on the rise. Woolf and Schoomaker (2019) cite worsening income inequality, socioeconomic pressures, and unstable employment as factors associated with increased mid-life mortality in the United States.

Unequal treatment

The Institute of Medicine landmark report, *Unequal Treatment: Confronting Racial and Ethnic Disparities in Health Care*, revealed that even when access to care and other issues that arise from differing socioeconomic conditions are accounted for, race and ethnicity remain significant predictors of the quality of health care received. The potential of the patient–provider relationship to perpetuate or ameliorate disparities in the quality of health care provided was highlighted (Smedley et al., 2003). Greater diversity among health care professionals, effective use of interpretation services, multidisciplinary care teams, and cultural diversity education and training were recommended both by *Unequal Treatment* and the Office of Minority Health's National Standards for Culturally and Linguistically Appropriate Services in Health and Health Care (CLAS) to reduce health disparities. Given that we are still far from reaching goals to reduce health disparities, the development of innovative approaches continues to be imperative (Villalobos et al., 2019).

Climate crisis and health

Life on Earth has been through five mass extinctions. We are in our sixth mass extinction and this one is human-caused (Ackerman, 2014). As a species, humans have survived seemingly insurmountable odds in our early beginnings and now number more than 7.7 billion people. Ironically, capitalism, the very economic system that has enabled some groups of people to live longer lives, has always been a threat to the health and existence of many racial and cultural groups, and now threatens the ongoing existence of all humans on Earth (Klein, 2015). By prioritizing exploitation and profits over caring for humankind and the living Earth, our extractive economic system has caused dangerous levels of global warming, extreme air and water pollution, desertification of once fertile lands, ocean acidification, and the tragic loss of humans, animals, and plant species. Although the heartbreaking loss of human lives is multiplied in the pandemic, the forced curtailment by the coronavirus of overproduction, overconsumption, and overtravel within capitalism has resulted in an astonishing cleansing of our common home (Milman, 2020).

Compounding one devastating problem with another, those most affected by climate change also face great catastrophes in the pandemic – particularly due to high levels of both poverty and air pollution in these nations (Wyns, 2020). People in poor countries, many of which are in the global south, have historically contributed the least to global warming, but have been disproportionately affected by climate change (Borunda, 2019). Prior to the pandemic, the extreme heat, pollution, natural disasters, variable rainfall patterns, water-borne diseases and diseases transmitted by infections were on the rise and had significant health consequences across the globe, but particularly affected communities in the global south (WHO, 2018) and communities of colour (NAACP, 2019). Access to the essentials for health – clean air, safe drinking water, sufficient food, and secure shelter – was increasingly jeopardized for millions of people as our planet warmed to unprecedented levels. Without the essential prerequisites for health and human needs prior to the pandemic, communities of colour and the global south have not had the capacity for a fair fight against the onslaught of COVID-19 (Wyns, 2020).

Indomitable people, our resilient planet, and their allies

Although the health consequences of oppression and the pandemic are dire, the struggle for health, health equity, and sustaining all life is momentous across the globe. Aware of their extreme vulnerability to amplified water stress and reduced agricultural yields prior to the pandemic, diverse African nations adopted grounding policies in agri-climate resilience (Dembele & Samuel, 2019) and African youth were organizing to fight for climate action (Mules, 2017). In defiance of negative health statistics, nine out of ten African American men, age 12 or older, currently don't use illicit drugs to numb the pain of their daily existence (National Center for Health Statistics, 2016). More than 50% of the 38,706 African American women participating in Boston University's Black Women's Health Study report that their physical and mental health is very good or excellent (Black Women's Health Imperative, 2019). Studies show that the lives of Black adults are at a disadvantage while they are young, with an increased risk of mortality. Yet when living past the age of 80, adults of African American heritage have a lower mortality rate than whites of a comparable age. If a person of African American heritage makes it to a certain ripe old age, their chance of longevity is high (Young, 2008). What does not kill a younger person of African American heritage makes them stronger as they grow into their lives as elders.

Positive health statistics illuminate the indomitable nature of human beings and can be found for every oppressed group. Remarkable statistics about improved air and water quality with the halt of capitalism illuminate the resilience of the Earth. Yet without large-scale efforts across the globe to transform capitalism and its multilayered systems of oppression into economic systems that place people and public health first, all life remains under threat. As Sharma et al. (2018) pointed out, educating practitioners regarding oppression and the social determinants of health alone does not translate into action against social and health inequity. Journal and discussion prompts and listening partnership questions in Table 9.2 invite the reader to increase their awareness of the impact of oppression on health and wellbeing. Listening partnerships will move the reader beyond merely learning statistics about the social determinants of health to connecting with peers about the devastating impact of oppression on health and wellbeing in their own lives and the lives of those for whom they care. They will also learn to support each other in battling feelings of discouragement about health disparities by identifying action steps they

TABLE 9.2 Partnerships for understanding the relationship between oppression, health, and wellbeing

Listening to understand racial and cultural identities and experiences with oppression	Questions for dialogue and connection Each speaker decides on which question(s) they would like to answer	Journal/discussion prompts
Oppression and health (15+ minutes each way)	What have you noticed regarding the social determinants of health in your family, friends, acquaintances, or people you have worked with? • Which health consequences of oppression for particular identity groups do you find the most moving, disturbing, or surprising? • What is your perspective on the oppression of males and do you agree that the societies we live in are oppressive towards boys and men, or not? • What does the wealth–health gradient mean for you personally? • What have you noticed or learned about climate change and health? How do you feel about it and what action would you like to take? • What helps you with feelings of discouragement? • Talk about resilience in yourself and others.	1. Complete the ACES Survey https://acestoohigh.com/got-your-ace-score/ and discuss or write in your journal about the meaning of your score. 2. Identify a racial or cultural group of which you would like to gain more knowledge and further explore the health challenges and health triumphs experienced by this group. 3. What action steps can you take to fight the health consequences of oppression?

can take towards health equity and justice. In Chapter 10, we will explore the process of building and strengthening alliances within and across racial and cultural lines as an essential step towards further dismantling oppression and achieving health and wellbeing for all humans and life on Earth.

References

Ackerman, D. (2014). *The human age: The world shaped by us.* New York: W. W. Norton & Company, Inc.

Black Women's Health Imperative, The (2019). *Indexus: What healthy Black women can teach us about health.* https://bwhi.org/wp-content/uploads/2020/01/BWHI_IndexUS_2019_Final-2.pdf

Borunda, A. (2019, April 22). Inequality is decreasing between countries: But climate change is slowing progress. National Geographic. www.nationalgeographic.com/environment/2019/04/climate-change-economic-inequality-growing/#close

Braveman, P., & Gottlieb, L. (2014). The social determinants of health: It's time to consider the causes of the causes. *Public Health Reports, 129*(1_Suppl. 2), 19–31. https://doi.org/10.1177/00333549141291s206

Davis, M. (2018, October 10). Nearly every country wants universal health care (except for one). Big Think. https://bigthink.com/politics-current-affairs/almost-everybody-wants-universal-healthcare

Dembele, D., & Samuel, S. (2019, May 25). Africa day: Pushing agri-climate justice to the policy level in Benin, The Gambia, and Kenya. Research Program on Climate Change, Agriculture and Food Security. https://ccafs.cgiar.org/blog/africa-day-pushing-agri-climate-justice-policy-level-benin-gambia-and-kenya#.XYaDFpNKjBJ

Edwards, F., Lee, H., & Esposito, M. (2019, August 20). Risk of being killed by police use of force in the United States by age, race–ethnicity, and sex. *Proceedings of the National Academy of Sciences of the United States of America, 116*(34), 16793–16798. https://doi.org/10.1073/pnas.1821204116

Halter, M. J., & Varcarolis, E. M. (2014). Understanding and managing responses to stress. In M. J. Halter (Ed.), *Varcarolis' foundations of psychiatric mental health nursing: A clinical approach* (7th ed., pp. 166–180). St Louis, MO: Elsevier/Saunders.

Klein, N. (2015). *This changes everything: Capitalism versus the climate.* New York: Simon & Schuster.

Mahler, D. G., Lakner, C., Aguilar, A. C., & Wu, H. (2020). The impact of COVID-19 (Coronavirus) on global poverty: Why Sub-Saharan Africa might be the region hardest hit. World Bank Blogs. https://blogs.worldbank.org/opendata/impact-covid-19-coronavirus-global-poverty-why-sub-saharan-africa-might-be-region-hardest

Malley, R., & Malley, R. (2020, March 31). When the pandemic hits the most vulnerable: Developing countries are hurtling toward coronavirus catastrophe. Foreign Affairs. www.foreignaffairs.com/articles/africa/2020-03-31/when-pandemic-hits-most-vulnerable

Marmot, M. (2017). The health gap: Doctors and the social determinants of health. *Scandinavian Journal of Public Health, 45*(7), 686–693. https://doi.org/10.1177/1403494817717448

McFarland, S. (2018, June 22). U.N. report: With 40M in poverty, U.S. most unequal developed nation. United Press International. www.upi.com/Top_News/US/2018/06/22/UN-report-With-40M-in-poverty-US-most-unequal-developed-nation/8671529664548/

McGibbon, E. (2012). *Oppression: A social determinant of health*. Black Point, Nova Scotia: Fernwood Publishing.

McGibbon, E., Etowa, J., & McPherson, C. (2008). Health-care access as a social determinant of health. *The Canadian Nurse, 104*(7), 23. https://pdfs.semanticscholar.org/5c71/0fa36567d84b8bbd957afcfd3bc2a469fd3e.pdf

Milman, O. (2020, April 2). Pandemic side-effects offer glimpse of alternative future on Earth Day 2020. The Guardian. www.theguardian.com/environment/2020/apr/22/environment-pandemic-side-effects-earth-day-coronavirus

Mules, I. (2017, December 11). COP23: African youth fighting for climate action. DW. www.dw.com/en/cop23-african-youth-fighting-for-climate-action/a-41333083

NAACP (2019). Environmental and climate justice. www.naacp.org/issues/environmental-justice/

National Center for Health Statistics (2016). *Health, United States, 2015: With special feature on racial and ethnic health disparities*. www.cdc.gov/nchs/data/hus/hus15.pdf#050

Office of Disease Prevention and Health Promotion (2019a). Social determinants of health. HealthyPeople.gov www.healthypeople.gov/2020/topics-objectives/topic/social-determinants-of-health

Office of Disease Prevention and Health Promotion (2019b). Disparities. HealthyPeople.gov www.healthypeople.gov/2020/about/foundation-health-measures/Disparities#6

Pickett, K. E., & Wilkinson, R. G. (2015). Income inequality and health: A causal review. *Social Science & Medicine, 128*, 316–326. https://doi.org/10.1016/j.socscimed.2014.12.031

Sharma, M., Pinto, A. D., & Kumagai, A. K. (2018). Teaching the social determinants of health: A path to equity or a road to nowhere? *Academic Medicine, 93*(1), 25–30. https://doi.org/10.1097/acm.0000000000001689

Smedley, B. D., Stith, A.Y., & Nelson, A. R. (2003). *Unequal treatment: Confronting racial and ethnic disparities in health care*. Washington, DC: The National Academies Press.

Tikkanen, R., & Abrams, M. K. (2020, January 30). U.S. health care from a global perspective, 2019: Higher spending, worse outcomes? The Commonwealth Fund. www.commonwealthfund.org/publications/issue-briefs/2020/jan/us-health-care-global-perspective-2019

Villalobos, A. V. K., Phillips, S., Zhang, Y., Crawbuck, G. S. N., & Pratt-Chapman, M. L. (2019, October). Oncology healthcare provider perspectives on caring for diverse patients fifteen years after *Unequal Treatment*. *Patient Education and Counseling, 102*(10), 1859–1867. https://doi.org/10.1016/j.pec.2019.04.030

Wilkinson, R. G., & Pickett, K. E. (2009). Income inequality and social dysfunction. *Annual Review of Sociology, 35*(1), 493–511. https://doi:10.1146/annurev-soc-070308-115926

Williams, D. R., Lawrence, J. A, & Davis, B. A. (2019) Racism and health: Evidence and needed research. *Annual Review of Public Health, 40*(1), 105–125 https://doi.org/10.1146/annurev-publhealth-040218-043750

Woolf, S. H., & Schoomaker, H. (2019). Life expectancy and mortality rates in the United States, 1959–2017. *Journal of the American Medical Association, 322*(20), 1996–2016. https://doi.org/10.1001/jama.2019.16932

World Health Organization (2017, December 13). World Bank and WHO: Half the world lacks access to essential health services, 100 million still pushed into extreme poverty because of health expenses. News release. www.who.int/news-room/detail/13-12-2017-world-bank-and-who-half-the-world-lacks-access-to-essential-health-services-100-million-still-pushed-into-extreme-poverty-because-of-health-expenses

World Health Organization (2018, February 1). Climate change and health. WHO factsheet. www.who.int/news-room/fact-sheets/detail/climate-change-and-health

World Health Organization (2019a). Working for better health for everyone, everywhere. www.who.int/about/what-we-do/who-brochure

World Health Organization. (2019b, July 15). World hunger is still not going down after three years and obesity is still growing – UN report. News release. www.who.int/news-room/detail/15-07-2019-world-hunger-is-still-not-going-down-after-three-years-and-obesity-is-still-growing-un-report

World Health Organization. (2019c, June 18). 1 in 3 people globally do not have access to safe drinking water – UNICEF, WHO. News release. www.who.int/news-room/detail/18-06-2019-1-in-3-people-globally-do-not-have-access-to-safe-drinking-water-unicef-who

World Health Organization (2019d, June 14). Drinking-water. WHO factsheet. www.who.int/news-room/fact-sheets/detail/drinking-water

World Health Organization (2019e). Health topics: Social determinants of health. www.who.int/social_determinants/sdh_definition/en/

Wyns, A. (2020, April 2). How our responses to climate change and the coronavirus are linked. World Economic Forum. www.weforum.org/agenda/2020/04/climate-change-coronavirus-linked/

Yancy, C. W. (2020, April 15). COVID-19 and African Americans. *Journal of the American Medical Association, 323*(19), 1891–1892. https://doi:10.1001/jama.2020.6548

Young, R. D. (2008). *African American longevity advantage: Myth or reality? A racial comparison of supercentenarian data* [Unpublished master's thesis]. Georgia State University. http://scholarworks.gsu.edu/gerontology_theses/10

10

PARTNERSHIPS TO DISMANTLE OPPRESSION

Dismantling oppression

Many lives will be saved, and human health will vastly improve as humans unite within and across racial and cultural lines to dismantle oppressive practices, policies, and structures in societies. It is always useful to remember that oppressive societies have only existed for 5% of human existence – roughly 10,000 of the 200,000 years that homo sapiens has inhabited the Earth. Though our tribal ancestors were violent towards each other, people did not systematically dominate, exploit, and mistreat each other as individuals or as groups until the advent of organized, agricultural societies. Despite the inherently loving and cooperative nature of humans, once the destructive and divisive forces of oppression took hold in these societies, it set the stage for increasing divisions that would profoundly impact human lives throughout the past ten millennia.

Through the partnerships of countless ordinary people living extraordinary lives, monumental efforts have been exerted and phenomenal gains have been made towards eliminating the subordination and systematic mistreatment of humans based on identities. The unity of great love, enduring tenacity, and brilliant minds have and will continue to undermine the inhuman and destructive forces that fuel oppression and threaten life on Earth. For our deepest yearning as humans is for a just and loving world and the flourishing of all life.

Finding our true humanity in each other

Despite our acts of inhumanity towards each other, the profound human tendency towards caring, empathy, and intelligent cooperation can be found – albeit sometimes buried deep beneath layers of hurt and conditioning that lead people to appear and act inhumanely towards each other. Listening to understand each other's experiences, to those who are targeted with oppression, and to those who are in roles as agents of oppression illuminates the reality that we are *all* damaged by oppression. To dismantle all forms of oppression, a tremendous amount of healing must occur between groups targeted with oppression and the groups acting as the agents of their oppression. Healing must also occur among the membership within groups targeted with oppression. Loving attention is necessary for the healing of *all* groups. This restorative kind of attention unleashes a deep and innate thriving life force within these groups and transforms their suffering which has resulted from being ripped apart from one another and separated from their innate goodness, worth, and dignity because of the viscous nature of oppression and internalized oppression.

Healing from internalized oppression within groups

VIGNETTE 10.1 GLORIOUS BLACK WOMEN – SISTAH LOVE: GLORYE NWA FI: RENMEN SÈ

As we learned in vignette 8.2, Angela, a Black nursing home social worker, yearned for the connection that only Black women could provide her. She missed having the deep healing conversations so necessary for her to thrive. She wondered if Mercy, a Haitian CNA, longed for that as well. Angela knew that to be close to Mercy required her (Angela) to embrace the truth – they both were descendants of enslaved Africans and shared common roots. Even though one was born in Maine, United States, and the other was born in Haiti, the white world treated them both as Black women. Her straight hair and light skin and Mercy's kinky hair and dark skin protected neither from the onslaught of white racism – disrespect, hate, and silencing. Angela knew that to thrive at work and in Maine, she needed Mercy in her life – together and forever. Sisters always.

Skilful, loving, and appreciative listening among members of groups targeted by oppression uproots internalized oppression and transforms it into pride and unity within those groups. With the many nuances of racially and culturally effective communication and loving relationships in place, as is exemplified by Angela and Mercy in vignette 10.1, self-hatred and self-loathing directed at oneself and one's own group are disarmed. The emotional release and processing of grief, fear, and indignation facilitate healing from internalized oppression as stories of vicious subjugation and injustice are shared and validated by trusted members of one's own group (Love, 2017). As we learned in previous chapters, the human mind heals from the scars of the mistreatment and is revitalized into its creative, loving, brilliant, and flexible essence in the presence of an aware individual or group of peers who can listen, love, and deftly lift spirits. The divisive and symbiotic forces of oppression and internalized oppression are undermined as people targeted by oppression are empowered and joined within groups to further the demise of all forms of humans harming humans.

VIGNETTE 10.2 HEALING SEPARATELY AND TOGETHER

As she developed friendships with People of Colour in her work as a nurse, Marcia became increasingly aware of the overt racism her friends experienced in their daily lives, and how sad and angry their stories made her feel. She also became increasingly aware of how bad she felt about the racism in her own family. Marcia joined the Ending Black Racism Team at work to learn to be a better ally to Black people. She was deeply moved by the generosity and love shown by Esther, the Black leader of the group, towards all people. Esther inspired the Ending Black Racism Team to engage in healing from the hurts of anti-Black racism and to take action to interrupt all forms of anti-Blackness in the workplace. Marcia was relieved when Esther directed the Black people, the other People of the Global Majority (PGM), and white people to meet separately some of the time, so each group could freely release emotions with each other about how anti-Black racism is affecting their particular identity group, and to learn how to challenge anti-Black racism in their daily lives.

Understanding that people only hurt others if they have been hurt can transform our perceptions of one another and facilitate the process of bridge-building and healing across lines (Brown & Mazza, 2005). This awareness is evident in rap superstar Jay-Z's response to derogatory comments that Donald Trump made towards immigrants from Haiti, El Salvador, and African nations. Jay-Z stated, "Donald Trump is a human being, too, somewhere along his lineage, something happened to him. Something happened to him and he's in pain and he's expressing it in this sort of way" (Wang, 2018).

Healing from the oppressor role as allies

People in oppressor roles benefit immensely from healing from the societal conditioning that forces them into inhuman roles (DiAngelo, 2018). For example, although men play oppressive roles towards women, no man asks to be in that role, but society coerces them into this role. Similarly, white people are forced into the role of oppressor towards People of the Global Majority, able-bodied people enact an oppressive role towards people with disabilities, hierarchies in health care place people in oppressor roles over other team members, and so on. The damage that occurs to people in the oppressor role is often obscured to people in that role. This damage could only occur because of a deep separation between people who are targeted with oppression and people in oppressor roles (DiAngelo, 2018). The awareness of the past and present realities of targeted groups for people in the oppressor role is distorted by misinformation that is shrouded in the enticement and illusion of power, control, and superiority over targeted groups. This is seen as their birthright. Thus, people in the oppressor role are separated from their own humanity and are often unaware of their own privilege and of the everyday threats to and persistent targeting of oppressed groups. In fact, they often feel victimized by the people they oppress – white people feel victimized by People of Colour, men feel victimized by women, parents feel victimized by their children, etc.

As we saw with Marcia in vignette 10.2, there is a tremendous relief in being with loving peers who share a particular oppressor conditioning and are jointly and persistently recovering from the damaging consequences of being in this dehumanizing role. This process assists people in oppressor roles in shedding guilt, fears, tears of grief and indignation as they reclaim their goodness, their loving connection to their innate selves and their people, and their ability to harness the power to right the wrongs of oppression (Jackins and others, 2002). The hurt human is released from oppressor conditioning and an increasingly effective ally emerges.

Allyship

VIGNETTE 10.3 HE CAN WASH HIS OWN GENITALS: MAAARI NIYANG HUGASAN ANG KANYANG SARILING MGA MASELANG BAHAGI NG KATAWAN

Grace, a young Pilipino CNA, and Janine, an older white OT, had a loving and trusting friendship. Grace came to Janine one day in tears, telling Janine that one of her older white male clients had asked her to wash his privates. Janine was outraged and stated, "You come and get me anytime any client asks you to wash their privates and I will set things straight." Janine entered the man's room and saw that he was feeding himself independently. Her quick OT assessment indicated that if he could feed himself, he could wash his own genitals and she artfully communicated this to the patient. Janine vented her indignation about this situation with Grace and other white women friends who shared her indignation. They had hearty laughs together about her creative approach to handling the situation. Janine became known among all the CNAs as the ally who would take swift action on their behalf when situations like this arose.

As Janine brilliantly exemplifies in vignette 10.3, strong allyship is demonstrated by people in oppressor roles when they take action in the world to fight oppression while backing oppressed groups. Taking action accelerates healing and recovery among people in oppressor roles and increases the possibility for deep and trusting relationships within and across lines. These relationships serve as the foundation for exchanging stories of pain, liberation, and celebratory re-emergence. Releasing tears of joy, dispelling guilt, scorning fear, loaning confidence, remembering each other's goodness and brilliance emboldens the mutual struggle against the annihilating forces of oppression. Allies and people targeted by oppression then become co-conspirators in ending oppression. Ultimately, victory is assured and is manifested within the body, mind, heart, and soul through such partnerships.

Mistakes as allies: The exquisitely human journey towards liberation

While many mistakes towards oppressed groups occur on an institutional level, people in oppressor roles also make *and* need to make umpteen mistakes in their interactions and relationships with people targeted by oppression in order to deepen relationships and become ever-stronger allies. This is evident in the many struggles and impasses experienced between men and women, white people and People of the Global Majority, heterosexual people and LGBTQ+ people, able-bodied people and people with disabilities, etc. People in oppressor roles can be made aware of their mistakes either by people targeted by their oppression or by their own people who can uphold their goodness while lovingly insisting that they:

- recognize and acknowledge their mistakes
- tell the whole truth
- heal the damage within themselves that caused the mistake
- apologize for the mistake and the harm done to others
- offer restitution or reparations
- make amends.

The non-linear process of rectifying mistakes is demonstrated in the magnificent work of Truth and Reconciliation Commissions around the world (Carnegie Council, 2015) and has an integral place in everyday interactions within and across lines as we listen, love, and lift spirits.

The significance of partnerships to dismantle racism

While the struggle to end every form of oppression is imperative, the work of dismantling racism, particularly anti-Black racism, appears to fuel the greatest progress towards creating a just and sustainable world for all life. Institutionalized racism, especially racism towards all people of African heritage, has destroyed and damaged the lives of hundreds of millions of people through slavery, colonization, apartheid, and racial discrimination, and continues to inflict large-scale damage towards People of Colour or People of the Global Majority across the globe (Jackins and others, 2002). Every human is deeply damaged by the presence of racism targeting Black-skinned people of the world, and every movement to create a better world is stalled by the divisive nature of institutionalized anti-Black racism (Jackins and others, 2002). Hence, the formation of healing partnerships to subvert all forms of racism is key to transforming all racial and cultural lines.

Healing within and across racial and cultural lines

Table 10.1 "Partnerships to build alliances and pride within and across racial and cultural lines" and Table 10.2 "Partnerships for deeper and restorative connections and understanding" provide questions that can light the path towards dismantling internalized oppression and oppressor patterns by supporting engagement not only within racial and cultural identity groups, but also across those groups. Given the depth of hurt experienced by people targeted by oppression and of those acting as an agent of oppression, engaging with listening partners or a small group of skilled listeners on a regular basis is necessary to heal the scars of our mistreatment and liberate human power, brilliance, and love.

It is incumbent upon people in oppressor roles to ask people targeted with oppression whether or not they want to hear stories of how they were conditioned to become an oppressor and/or acted on that conditioning. For example, females may not want to hear males share stories of sexism, People of the Global Majority may not want to hear white people share stories of their racism, and people with disabilities may not want to hear stories of ableism. This may only be appropriate when a depth of safety and caring has been realized between people targeted with oppression and those in oppressor roles. Leadership that transforms divisions among humans, whether in pairs, groups, or organizations, is often required for this level of safety and care to be attained. When this is achieved, our common humanity is powerfully revealed to each other as we mutually heal from the damage of oppression and seek our birthright – working as comrades in getting the world right. Chapters 11 and 12 will address leadership that transforms racial and cultural lines by listening, loving, and lifting spirits.

Journal/discussion prompts

Engage in listening partnerships on pp. 122–126 before completing these journal/discussion prompts.

1. What did you learn about yourself that you did not know before these listening partnerships?
2. What did you learn from your partner(s) that will assist you in becoming an even more powerful ally to your own people or people of _____ heritage?
3. What are you looking forward to in your partnerships with _____ _____?

TABLE 10.1 Partnerships to build alliances and pride within and across racial and cultural lines

Engaged listening to build alliances and pride within and across lines (15 minutes minimum each way on a selected identity)	Questions for dialogue and connection across all divisions (Members within constituency groups as well as allies across constituency groups will benefit from exchanging listening to the following questions. Speakers choose which questions they would like to address)
Strengthening natural alliances across gender Women and girls as warriors Men and boys as close brothers Transcending boundaries – Transgender, Intersex, Queer people, and your particular gender identity **Collaborating with people of diverse sexual orientation** Lesbians at the centre Gay men – whole and complete Full inclusion of Bisexual people Heterosexuals as allies to LGBTQ+ people **Embracing religions** Cherished and esteemed Muslims Vital and loved Jewish people Warm and welcoming Christians Your particular religious/spiritual group as a healing force Valued atheists and agnostics **Shedding class divisions** Proud and brilliant raised poor/working- class world changers Proud and visible middle-class agents of change	• What is magnificent about being _____? What is the truth about how phenomenal you are? • What are you proud of about being _____? • What has been hard/difficult about being _____? • How have you been mistreated as a _____? • What barriers have you had (or do you have) to overcome to have a great life as a _____? • Where has _____ oppression impacted your life? • How has internalized oppression impacted your life? • What is important for me to know about your life story? (Encourage us to feel grief, terror, confusion, self-doubt, and rage in telling our life story. Be open, interested, and eager to hear our triumphs and our hurts.) • What are you really like when _____ people are not around? What is it like to not have _____ around? • What can _____ people do for you that would have the most immediate impact on your life? • How can _____ people be your most trustworthy ally? • What is the most important thing you need to say to _____ people right now? • What do you think that _____ people do not understand about being a _____ person?

- What do you want others to know about _____?
- How have you been an ally to people from constituency groups other than your own?

Fully human owning class people

Treasuring the human race

Beautiful and courageous people of African heritage

Beloved and resilient people of Native/Indigenous heritage

Caring, unified, and compassionate people of Pacific Island and Pilipino heritage

Delightful and wise Arab people

Dignified and loving Asian heritage people (East, West, South, Central)

Enduring and powerful people of Latino/a heritage

Good white European heritage people

Universal humans – Multi-racial heritage people

Loving humans across their life span

Parents as shapers of a loving world

Powerful young people

Young adults as a key force

Bold older people

Honouring all shapes and abilities

Elegant and essential people with disabilities

Large and luscious people of size

Mental health system and emotional trauma survivors

Valiant navigators of recovery

Celebrating national origin and ethnicity

Glorious people of every ethnicity/national origin

Unwavering and strong migrants, asylum seekers, and refugees

TABLE 10.2 Partnerships for deeper and restorative connections and understanding

Engaged listening to transform racial and cultural lines	*Potential listening partnership questions* *Each speaker decides on which questions they would like to answer* *(15 minutes minimum each way on selected questions)*	*Discussion/journal prompts*
Gender	• Tell your life story as a male or female or as someone who did not or does not fit within binary gender identities. • Talk about your experiences as someone of your gender. • Share your vision of a world without gender oppression.	1. What is it like to have a dialogue about gender? 2. What is it like to be close to people of your own gender identity and people of other gender identities? 3. What do you think about the reality that there is no limit to the many creative ways of expressing ourselves as gendered beings?
Sex and sexual orientation	• While you were growing up, what attitudes were communicated to you about sex and sexual orientation by family, clergy, teachers, and friends? Were you able to talk openly with anyone? • Share your experiences with people of diverse sexual orientations. • If you feel comfortable doing so, talk about your experiences as someone of your sexual orientation.	4. What is it like to be close to people of your own sexual orientation? 5. If you have a friend who is LGBTQ+, what would it be like to ask them what it has been like to be his or her identity?
Class background	• Discuss your own class background. What did your parents and grandparents do for work? Did your family have enough, less than enough, or more than enough? Did your class background change? • What are your earliest memories of noticing that someone had less than enough or more than enough? • Discuss if you have interrupted classism.	6. Discuss your feelings about talking about class and the feelings you have about classism. 7. Discuss your vision of a world where everyone has their basic needs met. 8. What would it be like to give up your privilege?

Disability
- Talk about a disability you currently have or an accident, injury, or disability you had in the past. Describe both positive and challenging aspects of your situation.
- Share your experiences, both positive and challenging, with people with disabilities.

9. What disability would be the hardest for you to have or to work with and why?
10. If you are able-bodied, discuss what it is like or how you would like to reach out and build friendships with people with disabilities.

Race
- Talk about your early memories of noticing people with a skin colour different from your own.
- How has racism affected you?
- What have you done to interrupt racism?
- What is it like to follow the lead of People of the Global Majority?
- If you are white, what is it like to get close to other white people who are overtly racist?

11. What is it like to have a dialogue about racism?
12. Share your vision of a world without racism.
13. What are your committed action steps towards dismantling racism?
14. Discuss what action steps you think white people should take towards making reparations for the enslavement of African Heritage people.
15. Discuss any mistakes you have made in getting close to people of a different race. Discuss the support needed to learn from these mistakes.

Size
- What do you appreciate about your own body?
- What factors limit your ability to completely appreciate your body and the bodies of others?
- Share thoughts about how to interrupt oppression based on size.

16. Discuss whether large women and men feel comfortable talking with you about their oppression.
17. What would help you appreciate your own body more?

Age
- Have you ever been mistreated for being a particular age?
- Talk about the age group you have the hardest time relating to and share your experiences with that group.

18. What concerns you about growing older?
19. How would you like to be treated as an elder?

(continued)

TABLE 10.2 (Cont.)

Engaged listening to transform racial and cultural lines	Potential listening partnership questions Each speaker decides on which questions they would like to answer (15 minutes minimum each way on selected questions)	Discussion/journal prompts
Mental health	• What is your earliest memory of someone being described as crazy? • People are often labelled crazy when they have big feelings about the trauma and mistreatment they have endured. Discuss what you have noticed about this situation. • If you have received mental health services, what has been helpful, and what has not been helpful?	20. People who use mental health services are often stigmatized, jailed, homeless, and shunned by society. Discuss your awareness and experiences of this group that is often marked for destruction by society. 21. What have you noticed about human resiliency and the potential to recover from heavy trauma?
Religion/spiritual beliefs and heritage	• Describe your religious/spiritual heritage and current practices. • What are the strengths? Is there anything you wish was different about your religious heritage? • What has it been like to develop relationships with people of other religious/spiritual backgrounds?	22. What do you want to know about other religions or spiritual practices?
National origin and ethnicity	• Describe your ethnicity(ies) and national origin(s). • If you are not residing in your country of origin, why did you or your people locate to where you live now? • What is uniquely important that is offered by people of your ethnicity(ies) or national origin(s)? • Discuss if you are living on stolen land. If you are living on Native land, how have your people personally benefitted from the genocide of Native/Indigenous people?	23. Discuss the pros and cons of assimilation into a new culture or nation. 24. Discuss what it would be like or steps you might take to further explore your national origin(s) and ethnicity. 25. Discuss what action steps you think should be taken to make reparations to Native/Indigenous people for stealing their land and resources.

Adapted from: Froehlich, J. (2017), pp. 108–109.

References

Brown, C. R., & Mazza, G. J. (2005). *Leading diverse communities: A how to guide from healing to action* (Revised ed.). San Francisco, CA: Jossey-Bass.

Carnegie Council (2015, February). Examining the potential for an American Truth and Reconciliation Commission. Carnegie Council for Ethics in International Affairs. www.carnegiecouncil.org/publications/ethics_online/0102

DiAngelo, R. (2018). *White fragility: Why it is so hard for white people to talk about racism.* Boston, MA: Beacon Press.

Froehlich, J. (2017). Effective communication. In K. Jacobs & N. MacRae (Eds), Occupational therapy essentials for clinical competence (3rd ed., pp. 99–132). Thorofare, NJ: SLACK, Inc.

Jackins, T. and others (2002). *Working together to end racism: Healing from the damage caused by racism.* Seattle, WA: Rational Island Publishers.

Love, B. (2017). *Understanding and healing the effects of internalized racism: Strategies for Black liberation.* Seattle, WA: Rational Island Publishers.

Wang, A. (2018, January 28). Jay-Z thinks Trump is 'in pain.' The president responded by bragging about helping Black people. *Washington Post.* www.washingtonpost.com/news/politics/wp/2018/01/28/jay-z-thinks-trump-is-in-pain-the-president-responded-by-bragging-about-helping-black-people/

PART IV

Garnering love, hope, and leadership for human and planetary health

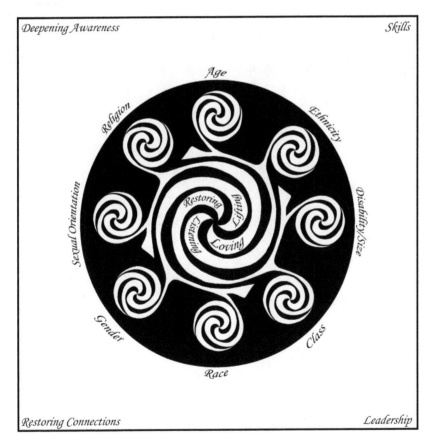

Deepening Awareness   Skills

Age

Religion

Ethnicity

Sexual Orientation

Disability/Size

Restoring
Listening
Loving
Gifting

Gender

Class

Race

Restoring Connections   Leadership

FIGURE 11.1 A model for transforming racial and cultural lines in health and social care

PART IV MODEL COMPONENTS LEADERSHIP: FACILITATION ACTIONS TO TRANSFORM HEALTH FOR ALL HUMANS AND THE PLANET

- modelling integrity, courage, caring, and decisive action
- inspiring hope, furnishing confidence, and communicating a shared vision for better health and wellbeing for all
- eliciting the thinking of groups to liberate creative ideas and develop best policies and practices
- committing to group goals, policies, and practices
- promoting listening exchanges to facilitate healing and unity within and across all racial and cultural lines
- supporting appreciations of all health team members, including oneself, and the planet
- collaborating to develop and implement action steps that lift spirits
- inviting constructive feedback to optimize collaborative efforts
- infusing enjoyment and playfulness in collaborative endeavours

11

HOPES AND VISIONS FOR HUMAN AND PLANETARY HEALTH

Voices of frontline workers as leaders

Voices of health and social care practitioners

Health and social care practitioners and all members of health teams are frontline workers in the struggle to promote health and wellbeing. Their voices are crucial to the process of transforming health and social care systems so that more and more lives can be saved and the health and wellbeing of all can be achieved. In this chapter, practitioners from diverse backgrounds share stories of pride in their work and challenges that interfere with optimal health and social care. Perspectives on the importance of the healing generated through engaged listening, a loving presence, and the artful lifting of spirits are shared. Stories of the transformative power of effective communication within and across racial and cultural lines, interprofessional collaboration, and leadership are highlighted. Hopes, wishes, and visions for health and social care systems that support the health and wellbeing of individuals, populations, communities, and the planet are presented.

The following excerpts from interviews with a variety of practitioners honour their experiences and perspectives. Their full credentials and place of employment can be found in the Acknowledgements section. While we are delighted to elevate the voices of a variety of health and social care practitioners, we acknowledge and honour the work of all members of health and social care teams, many of whom are not represented in the excerpts below. The reader is invited to enjoy learning from the practitioners who are represented in our interviews, and to engage in ongoing listening, loving, and lifting spirits with diverse members of the health and social care teams and to share the gifts of who they are with each other. Listening partnership questions and journal/discussion prompts in Table 11.1 can be used not only with listening partners, but with all health and social care practitioners encountered in one's daily life. As we deepen connections, learn from each other, and heal together from the hardships of our work and our daily lives, we clarify our vision and path towards human and planetary health and wellbeing. The voices of practitioners are also integrated into Chapter 12 as we explore inherent and designated leadership – leadership that transforms experiences in health and social care to save lives and improve health and wellbeing for all cultural and racial groups and the planet.

What are you proud of and appreciate about being a _____ and about your profession as a whole?

> **Carl, PA** – The opportunity and the ability to provide care and the commitment to service.
>
> **Islane, RN, MSN** – To me, it is a privilege to be a nurse, and especially a mental health nurse. I meet people where they are and most of the time, in their worst times. I can be with them on their journey and use my nursing skills to give them hope to fight back.
>
> **Joshua, MS, OT** – You share a particular bond with clients because you work on such meaningful things in a creative way that resonates with just them.
>
> **Kelli, MSW** – We have a wide view of the world. I love being with kindred spirits who are also social workers who see the world the way I do. It's a calling for me. I appreciate I found where I belong.
>
> **Marie, MSW** – When facilitating life stories, we bring pertinent information to the team so they see the clients in the context of their environment and their lived experiences and history. I think this brings a lot of empathy and contributes to better care. As social workers, we get paid for being really caring – and that's great.
>
> **Patricia, BS, OT** – I am proud of being able to come up with creative ways to motivate patients and to connect with them – especially those patients who are having a difficult time adjusting to their conditions or situations. I have to get very creative.
>
> **Regina, MSW** – I love helping individuals become more confident and independent, and advocating on the individual, community, and societal level.
>
> **Sabine, Cultural Broker** – I love helping people, seeing the joy in clients' faces, and solving problems.
>
> **Said, OTD** – I am proud of occupational therapy's holistic approach to improving people's mental and physical conditions in order to improve their lives. It is an honor to be a professor teaching new practitioners who are helping people, throughout the age span, live their lives fully. I am also very proud and honoured that I am helping to bring occupational therapy to Morocco, the country I am originally from. I can be called the "Father of OT in Morocco".
>
> **Saige, Tribal Youth Engagement Manager** – I am really honoured to be able to work with the youth – being able to help, to support them in leadership roles, and to uplift their voices.
>
> **Steve, DPT** – When you're seeing clients, they are debilitated and weak and are often functioning well below their baseline, and at times feel hopeless.

Being a PT affords me an opportunity to not only play the role of a therapist, a teacher, and a counsellor to patients, family members, and caregivers. I come away each day knowing I made a small difference in people's lives.

Usha, MD – I enjoy getting to know about the lives of patients and piecing together their stories into a cohesive history. I love addressing the root cause of their disease and helping them live healthier and have a better quality of life.

What is hard, difficult, or challenging about being a _____?

Carl, PA – I went from clinical practice to public health, to academia, and now do consult work. As a PA, you are trained and educated in the medical model. PA education is a modified form of medical school. They literally took four years of medical school and squeezed it down to two and a half years. You are held to a single standard of excellence relative to clinical knowledge and clinical skills. At the same time, you must come to grips with the fact [that] no matter how good you are and how good you get, you will never be captain of the team. You find yourself having to constantly temper your own ego and your own assertiveness and to subsume it for the benefit of the team. Also, people are still asking what a PA is. We have done a really poor job of answering that question.

Islane, RN, MSN – I want to make everybody happy, give health back, but I am not always able to. Sometimes just being there is all I can do.

Joshua, MS, OT – As culturally fluid and as culturally sensitive as I thought I was, I still was never as informed as I wanted to be – I have to learn from my mistakes.

Kelli, MSW – It's easy for other people to dismiss the experience of other human beings in a way we can't. It feels never-ending and often feels like the problems are so systemically focused. Lots of things break my heart because of all the tragedy we see, and all the injustice and unfairness in the world I can't look away from.

Marie, MSW – There are more complicated situations and multiple co-occurring stressors that people are facing. There are waning resources or no resources at all with the expectation that we're supposed to bring some resources when all we can bring is listening, validation, and witnessing the struggles. We shed light on people's resilience. There is also a conflict from wanting to create social change within a broken system that is designed to keep things status quo. Social work is primarily a female-dominated profession and we are undervalued and often expected to be self-sacrificing.

Patricia, BS, OT – Waking up in the morning and gearing up for whatever racial or other discriminatory incidents might come at others or myself, and knowing I am on my own and don't have any support is challenging for me as an OT. People may sympathize, but actions to mitigate these occurrences, especially if they are coming from patients, do not seem to exist. When the racist statements come from people in positions of power it makes it even more difficult to challenge due to fear of retribution. I was lucky in one situation where a fellow therapist was discussing lynching in the presence of his patient and mine. I asked him to stop as it was not appropriate, especially with an elderly Black woman who most likely had experienced much of that type of hatred over her years. He did not stop. I escorted his patient and mine back to their rooms and then reported it to the Rehab Director and Administrator. He was terminated from his position on that day. It was the only time over my 25 years of being an OT that action had been taken that I am aware of. There are so many racial incidents on the job that documenting all of those will take another full-time job. The exhausting fight for your right to be treated with respect as a person and as a professional is what makes it challenging about being a Black OT.

Sabine, Cultural Broker – Understanding two cultures. Some stuff is okay in America, and some stuff is okay in my community (the Democratic Republic of the Congo). Finding a balance can be hard. It is difficult to explain to Americans what "okay" is back home.

Said, OTD – Many people still don't know what occupational therapy is. For example, when some patients mistakenly call me a physical therapist, I take the time to gently correct them because I know this contributes to people understanding the important role occupational therapy can play in their wellness.

Saige, Tribal Youth Engagement Manager – Not much has changed around racism. When youth share stories about racism and microaggressions within the schools, it hurts my heart to hear their stories.

Steve, DPT – Working with patients and/or family members who aren't entirely invested in the recovery of the patient is hard and can be frustrating. Another challenging aspect of having a job in rehabilitative medicine is the huge focus on productivity to the point, at times, it feels like it's just about the bottom line. I changed careers to move away from billable hours, but have come to a realization and acceptance [that] it is what it is, any job will have its challenges, and this is no different. With that said, I love what I do, and this job allows me to serve others in a way that embraces my passion for health.

Share about another health or social care profession you have appreciated collaborating with

Carl, PA – I don't want to sound trite, but I appreciate collaborating with all professions with no exception. Cognitively and legally, PAs are tied at the hip with physicians, but we collaborate very closely with nursing, therapy, and everyone else. Because of the philosophy of the profession and the team model in which we are trained, we come to respect pretty much all of our colleagues. There is some tension between PAs and nurse practitioners. We may not be brothers and sisters, but we are first cousins, and I hope the competitiveness dies away.

Islane, RN, MSN – We are in this together. My role is not more important than any other role. A collaborative approach is what improves patient outcomes.

Joshua, MS, OT – Social work closely mirrors some of what OT does, and they are very receptive to the unique ideas of OT.

Kelli, MSW – Collaborating with my fellow interprofessional folks has just been the joy of my life – one of the most fun things.

Marie, MSW – Working on an interdisciplinary team is highly needed in hospice. Nurses often do pain relief and symptom management. In part, I help with psychological, emotional, and existential pain as families resolve conflict, find meaning, and mutual forgiveness around death and dying. The value of the team comes in as each discipline brings a different lens to our work.

Patricia, BS, OT – Social workers, nurses, and other disciplines being willing to work together is so important. I like that social workers really advocate for their patients.

Regina, MSW – I have appreciated working within the overall health care profession and collaborating on the state and local level.

Sabine, Cultural Broker – The local medical centre and some community dentists are helpful.

Said, OTD – I always look forward to collaborating with my peers. I work and collaborate at the clinical level or academic level with doctors, PTs, PT assistants, nursing [staff], speech therapists, social workers, and public health professionals. We have to collaborate to achieve clients' outcomes.

Saige, Tribal Youth Engagement Manager – A lot of collaboration happens whether it's with the youth departments, tribal organizations, tribal government, or outside of the tribal communities.

Steve, DPT – OTs and PTs are constantly talking to each other, working in concert through co-treatments and/or collaborating on functional goals to meet the needs of patients when they return home, [to] assisted living facilities, or other living arrangements. I've learned so much from the OTs I've worked with and really value their insight and expertise.

Usha, MD – Working with durable medical equipment companies for discharge planning and follow-up is so important – connecting all the pieces and making sure that treatment is completed, and the patient's home situation is able to support their needs.

What have you noticed about listening, loving, and lifting spirits as a student or as a health or social care practitioner?

Carl, PA – The philosophy of the PA profession is relationship-centred. Listening is probably the most important thing any clinician can do because if you listen carefully enough, the patient will tell you what the problem is and often will also tell you what the answer is. So, you can't hurry through patient encounters. Every person has a story to tell. Then you can be of service to them as their agent and advocate. You might not like every patient, but you have to love all your patients. My approach to lifting spirits is to be honest with my patients and to help them wherever their road leads them – to a complete cure or to the end of their lives. I tell patients I am on the journey with them and not to worry until I'm worried – then we're always in concert with one another. I try not to give my patients false hope, but I try to help them find whatever hope there is.

Islane, RN, MSN – Listening is the most important part. We listen with our eyes, ears, and heart. There is much we cannot express with words so we must listen with the heart, see and feel non-verbal communication. If we don't listen, how can we help? Of course, we love. You have to love the profession first to be able to love people on their journey. Caring is an important part of nursing theory. In my opinion, all the care teams, in general, should treat every patient with compassion. Nursing should collaborate with the team and ensure we are on the same page in terms of loving, listening, and lifting spirits.

Joshua, MS, OT – Listening is just huge, it's just so multi-faceted. If you listen it'll take you so much further within the profession than you could ever imagine. When you do care, the clients can feel the love you're providing them at that moment. Sometimes it's difficult with patients just because life is beating them down. If you can find a way to show them you like, care [for], and love them, I think then you can lift their spirits.

Kelli, MSW – Listening with an open heart is probably the most important thing I ever do. There is no word in the English language to describe that experience of being so intimate with someone who is not a child, a parent, a lover, or even a friend. It's a love that is indescribable in the context of that relationship. Clients begin to feel unburdened as they begin to feel heard. People feel less crazy, and I think that's the lifting. They become more self-aware, somewhat more open-hearted or they see what's around them more, and then they can't help but look after Mother Earth.

Marie, MSW – I know there are situations I walk into and mostly what I am doing is listening. As I leave, or a situation winds down, families will often say you're really good at what you do, and in my mind, I realize what I did was listen attentively and with compassion. A lot of people just need to tell their story and be heard.

Patricia, BS, OT – Listening is not just using your ears but is listening between the lines to decipher what someone is saying or not saying. Sometimes you do not have to decipher. Many times, people will tell you exactly what they are thinking, needing, or wanting.

Regina, MSW – I run a high from caring about others.

Sabine, Cultural Broker – To be able to listen, love, and lift spirits, you need to genuinely have a compassionate and loving heart, to be patient and understanding, and to always try to put yourself in the other person's shoes.

If we can all act like that, this world would truly be a better place. I've always been a great listener. It's not difficult. In my culture, women keep quiet. We are listeners. In caring for people from my country, I know what people have been through. I have been there.

Said, OTD – Listening is the most important thing for health care professionals. If you approach your clients with respect, are open and honest with your intentions, and how you are being, they trust you and are more willing to participate in therapy and trust the OT process. You can't practise something if you don't love it, especially when you are working with people who are vulnerable physically and mentally. Humour never hurts. It's frequently been my way with clients, to make a joke at my own expense, and bring some joy and levity to their challenging situation. I try to treat everyone the same, but sometimes I see where some people need more support. If a patient does not speak a language I know, I learn three or four words of their language and share it with them. It shows I care. Their eyes get bigger, it catches their attention and makes a connection. I show them I care about them.

Saige, Tribal Youth Engagement Manager – Sometimes it's hard because I want to solve and fix everything, but no, there is a lot of just listening, showing up, and being consistent. I'm also kind of like their Auntie, just with healthy boundaries, showing love and support.

Steve, DPT – I think initially when I first started working with patients, I had a tendency to talk too much and not listen enough. I've learned [that] patients' commitment to a care plan requires they need to be heard, so you build that connection and trust which leads to better patient participation and commitment. At times I just remind myself it's okay sometimes to keep quiet and listen, so I can make sure the things I'm wanting for my patients are aligned to what the patients are hoping to achieve in the long term.

Usha, MD – It is important I take care of myself and my emotions first. When I have addressed my own needs, I find it is easier to be mindful and be in the present, so I am available to truly listen to my patients.

What have you noticed about listening, loving, and lifting spirits within and across racial and cultural lines?

Carl, PA – I set up the Center for Transcultural Health at UNE. A question that I would ask myself and help my colleagues and students address when we were dealing with cultural differences is how we can be of help to someone who has a different worldview and possibly a different set of health beliefs than our own. How can we keep not just the difference between us apparent, but undertake the effort to understand who they are, what they believe, and not impose our personal, medical, or social belief system on them?

Islane, RN, MSN – It is a culture shock to be in the US. I come from a religious culture and people care more about each other and help each other. Family means extended family and close friends or even your neighbour.

We take care of people with different values and beliefs – we need to respect their values even if it differs from yours. It is not always easy. In my culture, we have no boundaries when it comes to caring. Here you set boundaries. When lifting spirits in my culture, we use religion and faith a lot. Here, people don't even want to talk about religion. People find resilience from religious beliefs/faith. It's a protective barrier.

Joshua, MS, OT – Some of those hiccups come because people are very afraid to ask just because they don't want to seem ignorant. It is difficult to navigate loving and caring because you just are unsure of where those boundaries are. I know being ignorant, unaware, and in the dark is also harmful and offensive. If you listen, you can see where the love needs to be and uplift your client's spirits in that way.

Kelli, MSW – I grew up in a very racially diverse area, but [I] don't think I ever really had much appreciation for the experience of People of Colour in my life – we were taught to be colourblind. When I moved to Maine, I did home-based counselling with people on a small island, and although they were white, I didn't understand their dialect. It was a moment of learning that culture doesn't necessarily mean just race, ethnicity, or where somebody comes from – culture is also about community. The same thing happened when I worked with French Catholic people. I was raised Irish Catholic, but I was taken aback because I knew nothing about their culture – I had to be open-hearted and listen, and not make assumptions.

Marie, MSW – Understanding cultural differences and not imposing my lens, assumptions, or generalizations is significant. I've learned to take my cues from interpreters and cultural brokers – there are some questions I've learned not to ask, and particular words I've learned not to use. Sometimes when the interpreter is in another room, there is eye contact and non-verbal communication. There is a human connection beyond words that elevates us and lets us be human with each other around deep grief and loss.

Patricia, BS, OT – Medically, patients are in the hospital for a reason, but I always find a way to connect with people of different races and cultures. Here in Minnesota, there are many Swedish, Norwegian, and people from different African nations, so I still have to find a way to connect with them and lift spirits. Even if I am not from their background, I learn a few words or phrases of their language or find interesting facts or traditions of their nationality and try my best to bring it to them at the facility.

Regina, MSW – Listening, loving, and lifting spirits within and across racial and cultural lines is why I do this work. It is exhausting because discrimination is alive and well in America. I am more aware of that than anything else. I ran refugee services – those are the folks who are the reason I am a social worker. I have a deeper connection with them than anyone else. Yet, I also found I wanted to help the poor white client as much as I wanted to help the poor Black client. Poor is poor.

Sabine, Cultural Broker – Across cultural and racial lines, other people are not good at listening. I had to accept that. There is nothing I can do to change it. Living with that is not easy. We have to learn how to live. I comfort my people by sharing my experience. I explain to my people where I am today and encourage them to keep faith that someday it will be okay. Praying is a huge part of my culture. Loving across cultural and racial lines is very difficult. Not all white people are bad – some white people are nice.

Said, OTD – I come from Morocco, a diverse culture known for people helping one another, the land of generosity. Moroccans like to feed you, invite you into their home, and do little things to please you. It is in my DNA. I try to use my heritage and those traits in the things I do to connect with others who have a different culture or heritage than me. Being sensitive to other people's cultures and backgrounds is very important since we OT practitioners serve a diverse population.

Saige, Tribal Youth Engagement Manager – I didn't grow up within any of the tribal communities in Maine. I'm Yakama. It took a while to build relationships within the tribal communities in Maine. We're building resilience and connection and it crosses lines. I can sit, listen, and hear that tradition and culture is everything. It's in everything we do and it is a resilience factor – it's prevention. It's a protective barrier. Connection and culture is prevention. We're sharing the traditional language with the youth and we're incorporating tradition and ceremony within the things we do.

Steve, DPT – I can probably count on one hand how many People of Colour I worked with while I was a PT in the Midwest. Since moving out to California last summer, I've noticed my caseload has completely changed where more than 50% of the patients I serve are now People of Colour. One thing I've observed since being out West is [that] it does seem Asian families tend to have a greater sense of obligation when it comes to taking care of their elders and sick family members. This is not true across the board, but generally speaking, that's what I've noticed when I'm treating patients of various ethnicities and races; there seems to be a very strong commitment and participation amongst the family members – consequently, they are very involved in the care of their loved ones. This can be a benefit when you need extra eyes and hands to help a patient recover safely, but can also be a drawback if family members are overbearing and not able to see or accept instruction or feedback to best help a patient.

Usha, MD – I think it is important [for] both parties involved in the conversation to set aside their intrinsic bias and preconceived notions and inconsequential issues before they can connect at a truly human level.

Discuss your perspective on the role of having others (peers, therapists, colleagues, partners) listen, love, and lift your spirits in your role as a _____

Carl, PA – Well, I certainly have my wife, and I have been fortunate to always have one or two close friends I could be totally open and candid with. Periodically, I have used professional resources.

Joshua, MS, OT – I believe my own success as an OT comes from having people there to listen, love, and uplift my spirits. I am beyond fortunate to have a support system that genuinely cares about my wellbeing, affording me the luxury to continue providing patient-centred care.

Kelli, MSW – This reminds me of the song from *The Lion King*, "the Circle of Life". In order to move forward with passion and commitment to work on behalf of vulnerable people, hold hope for the world, and maintain my spiritual and emotional centre, I must find and be open to, trust, and accept support and love from colleagues, family, friends, and my therapist. Being isolated and feeling alone in the world can make life feel like a very dark and hopeless place. A social worker who feels hopeless is not good for anyone!

Marie, MSW – I think if listening to each other was a regular occurrence, burnout in frontline workers would be reduced. It would be beneficial to create a space where people can debrief, come together, and talk about our work. When I am listened to or loved or when there's a lot of validation and lifting spirits, it proves highly beneficial. I find for health care workers, a little bit of attention, support, validation, and resource has great value. It goes a long way. I think when people have a need to talk [and] when I actually listen with loving compassion and really try to reach for their greatest good, it has a trickle-down effect.

Sabine, Cultural Broker – Many people are not good listeners. Fortunately, my husband is a very good listener and listens well to me.

Share how your racial and cultural identity has influenced your practice

Carl, PA – It has made me more sensitive and able to engage in practice with different people. During much of my formative years, I was the only Black in my school or other situations. So, I clearly understood the minority/ majority kinds of situations and the misunderstandings [that] can occur. I was often the only Black professional in hospitals where I worked and in the communities I lived in. I knew how Black people in the North expected to be treated. When I went to the South, I quickly appreciated how in the South there is a different culture of Blackness and how people expected to be treated. I was sensitive to that. I had opportunities to understand the differences between being a majority and being in the minority. I expanded into international communities when I was a U.S. Army Medic in Vietnam. When working in local villages, I was often the only Black person and the only Westerner, so it gave me a lot of opportunities to learn cultural humility. I have not always been successful. When I failed, I failed famously, learning from those failures.

Islane, RN, MSN – As a Haitian woman, racial and cultural identity has lots of influence and challenges. We must be aware. Racism is right here. People notice my accent. Some people I would like to work with don't want to work with me because of my racial identity and accent.

Joshua, MS, OT – As a Peruvian man, I really pride myself on trying to be an advocate for those who can't speak up or choose not to speak up. Also, hanging out with more women as an OT student has shown me a different aspect of life I hadn't related to – I was not aware of some gender differences. The female point of view is just completely different than mine in many ways.

Kelli, MSW – Being Irish was a huge source of pride in my family. We were also working class – my dad worked in a paper mill. I come from hardy stock. But part of my identity is really about being a Jersey girl, having my deepest roots in New York City. I also identify with queer issues; I feel really passionate about equality and LGBTQ+ rights.

Marie, MSW – I've experienced the effects of classism and adversity in my life. Many loved ones struggle with addictions. What I have always found to be most helpful is when people suspend judgment. Addictions aren't an individual choice – it's a societal, systemic problem. I have a lot of compassion for people who are disenfranchised. As a Franco-American, I bring a cultural lens to my work because my people have a history of losing our language and being targeted for destruction. When I meet People of Colour in Maine, which is mostly a white state, and hear their stories of environmental and social inequities, my background enables me to find places where I related to their struggles and know it's not about them. It is a much bigger, systemic issue. It was probably worth all the thousands of dollars spent on social work school to learn about the social determinants of health and the ACE [Adverse Childhood Experiences] studies. I learned how so many problems aren't an individual responsibility but are caused by societal structures.

Patricia, BS, OT – I always have to go in and know clients may or may not connect with me as a Black female, but I still try to find a way. This is reality. My spirituality and upbringing have enabled me to look beyond the external shell and get to the crux of the issue. I was born and raised in Sierra Leone, West Africa until I was 8 years old. I was a proud Sierra Leonean. Sierra Leone is known as one of the most hospitable countries to foreigners despite her history of its people being ripped away from their home and forced into slavery in the United States. In other words, once I arrived here in the US, I became a Black person. I did not identify myself as Black until I came to the US. My value suddenly changed as a human being. Thank God for my grandmother who used to kneel down and pray with us, quoting Luke 23:34, "Then Jesus said, 'Father, forgive them; for they know not what they do'." My grandmother was a Sierra Leonean nurse and a Catholic who had wedded my German grandfather. We were taught to love and care for everyone. These early childhood values have influenced my practice.

Regina, MSW – As an African American woman, my passion is around the policy and systematic change. I enjoy that. I am fuelled by my passion for social justice.

Sabine, Cultural Broker – All people from my country (the Democratic Republic of the Congo); if I talk on their behalf, they feel comfortable, and more confident because I am from their country.

Said, OTD – I am a Muslim, and Islam calls for helping people, especially the vulnerable. I try to connect with clients, to be of service to them to make their lives better. At the end of my life, I will face my Maker and be held accountable for my actions. This pushes me to be the best occupational therapist, teacher, and advocate I can be. As a man of colour in America who was raised in a very racially diverse country, I feel I have insights available to help guide my practice with clients of colour. I've felt the sting of racism, intentional or not, subtle or explicit in my daily life, student life, and professional life. I know what it's like to be vulnerable, sick, in need of support in a system that does not see all of me or sees just the outside of me and makes assumptions about how my own health care should be directed. Therefore, I'm very vigilant to provide client-led care.

Saige, Tribal Youth Engagement Manager – As an Indigenous/Native woman, tradition and culture is everything. It's a resilience factor. It is prevention. It's a protective barrier. When we share the traditional language with youth and incorporate tradition and ceremony within the things we do, we build resilience.

Steve, DPT – Growing up in the Midwest, I was one of four or five Asians at all my schools, two of them were my siblings, so not much exposure to diversity in my formative years. I think I was a bit lost and just wanting desperately to fit in and not be judged by what I looked like. Unfortunately, I was running into a lot of racism, and because of that, I pushed away my Asian identity. At the time I really hated being Asian because of the hateful things it brought upon me. Later, in my high school years, I had an opportunity to go to summer school in Seoul, meeting other Korean Americans my age who were super proud of who they were and really embracing their ethnicity and culture. This was a moment of change for me and started a period of confusion, struggle, and self-reflection. These are things I still continue to sort out even today, and I think it makes me more empathetic, sensitive, and open to the racial and cultural differences amongst the patients I treat and colleagues I work with and this perspective serves me well in my practice.

Usha, MD – As an immigrant from India, I understand [that] despite all the camouflage, the fundamental human needs are the same. My childhood and upbringing have enabled me to look beyond the external shell and get to the crux of the issue.

Discuss your experiences with collaboration and leadership in your role as a _____

Carl, PA – Collaboration is critical as a PA. The physicians want something to occur on behalf of a patient and it's your job to make sure that happens and work with the other team members to bring that about. You have to achieve a sense of trust with the other people you engaged with, so they understand you respect and appreciate them. We did this well in the professional geriatric education programme. It was modelled on a horizontal hierarchy and the absolute need to collaborate. You had to understand what everyone else did, what their role expertise was, and what they brought to the table or bedside on behalf of the patient. It was far more advantageous for the patient that leadership is situational – the issue or problem would drive who would be the leader. We were ultimately successful, and it was a transformative experience for all. I've had leadership roles within my profession, and politically at state and national levels. I learned you have to have a clear vision and make goals others buy into. Leaders need to know what their skill sets are and find people who do the things they don't do well. Leaders cannot do it all. I am a good listener, a reasonably good communicator, and a good convenor who can bring people together. I can succinctly state back whatever complex set of issues people are fighting about and make it seem clear to people. I am a big picture guy.

Islane, RN, MSN – Collaboration is very, very important in health care. If we collaborate, we can see all the benefits for the patient. When we don't collaborate, the patient is the one who will suffer. They won't get the quality of care they deserve.

Joshua, MS, OT – The biggest part of collaboration is keeping the lines of communication open. Also, I build strong rapport so others have no problem being open with me because they know I'll take the feedback.

Kelli, MSW – I collaborated a lot with psychiatrists, medical doctors, and case managers. The hardest part is getting in touch with people. It's about making time and having the time. It is harder now because of productivity demands. Collaborating through the electronic health record is just crazy. As for leadership, my clinical social work skills really make it much easier to be a good leader by listening with an open heart.

Marie, MSW – Collaboration in homecare gives people a fuller picture of an individual or family. Our clients are better served. Collaboration has to occur at every level. I often lead from behind by encouraging co-workers to find their voice about their concerns in the workplace. I also interrupt lateral violence in the workplace. When team members say oppressive things about clients with addictions or obese clients, I help them put themselves in the shoes of our clients. I say let's just imagine that client's family member or loved one is sitting right here. Would you say those words?

Regina, MSW – I've been lucky to be able to collaborate with so many people and organizations around so many issues, including the police in a local city in developing a policy so [that] police don't promote any officer unless they have interviewed a refugee

Sabine, Cultural Broker – I work behind the scenes and challenge people to tell each other the truth. I have had good experiences collaborating with community health workers and case managers.

Said, OTD – I believe in the power of connection. I love networking, collaborating, and connecting people to like-minded people around the world. I'm fortunate to collaborate on projects that are national (i.e. Lymphedema Advocacy Group) and international (building OT in Morocco and other countries with no OT yet). Empowering other OT practitioners and students here in the USA and globally is a deep-rooted calling that is inherently part of my own professional identity. In fact, it's become a bit of a joke; when I go places, "You know everyone!" is the most frequent thing my family, students, and colleagues say to me. When you are in a role to constantly connect people you become a leader, intentionally or not. It's a gift given to me, for which I am grateful.

Saige, Tribal Youth Engagement Manager – A lot of collaboration happens. There is not one person deciding anything. It's equal – like we're on the same page. We hold space there.

Steve, DPT – I'm constantly collaborating every single day. Working as part of a team is absolutely mandatory in health care, because you're working with so many different disciplines, and ultimately, we're all trying to serve the best interests of the patients. Even if you're not a formal leader, you end up having to be a leader in providing patients, family members, and caregivers [with] the education, training, and consultation they need for the best recovery possible.

What has supported the process of giving and receiving feedback to support best practices?

Carl, PA – If I am doing what you want and expect me to do, let me know, but even more importantly, if I am not, it is absolutely critical you tell me. I cherish feedback, otherwise, I am lost. I try to deliver feedback in non-challenging ways.

Islane, RN, MSN – Receiving feedback from patients and co-workers is important. I appreciate it when someone tells me if I am not doing well. I like checking in with licensed nursing assistants (LNAs) and mental health technicians (MHTS) for positive or negative feedback. Feedback from the patient is always important. I use them to improve the care I'm providing and my approach as a nurse.

Kelli, MSW – Giving honest feedback is harder than receiving feedback for me. I have learned how to frame honest feedback in a way that's not too soft, doesn't miss the point, and is also easy to hear.

Marie, MSW – Feedback that matters to me is what I hear from families and patients either while they're still alive and with us or after they have died – knowing we did something, knowing there are places to improve or anything in between. I always make sure to pass along compliments of my co-workers to them and their supervisors.

Patricia, BS, OT – To motivate the staff and show appreciation, I carry around a stack of appreciation cards. Some days it is random, sometimes it is the first ten people I walk by. Everyone is working hard – they should be appreciated. Everyone is essential.

Regina, MSW – Nobody can fault you for being honest and telling the truth – but it depends on the relationship.

Sabine, Cultural Broker – It is easy to listen to feedback. It is common in my community. Americans don't like feedback. They get upset. I always give my feedback.

Said, OTD – I like immediate feedback on anything I am doing so right away I can adapt. [The] weekly peer review of documentation and treatments in a skilled nursing facility I worked in was a very successful model for me. It pushed me to be more creative, seek more evidence-based practice, and utilize my peers' feedback.

Saige, Tribal Youth Engagement Manager – Receiving and giving feedback is kind of ingrained because we are so collaborative. I'll always ask [for] feedback from the youth about how I could have done better.

Steve, DPT – In order to get better, you need to be receptive to asking for and receiving feedback. I know there will be personal weaknesses in myself I may not recognize. Therefore, I welcome opportunities from my peers, supervisors, and patients to hear critiques and not get defensive, just work to get better.

What concerns you most as a health or social care practitioner?

Carl, PA – Our health care system or the lack of it is the only thing that concerns me. We don't have a rational system in the US. Health care is one of the four pillars of society and we don't have it.

Islane, RN, MSN – Equity in health care. We need to improve cultural awareness and cultural competencies to provide equitable care and give everybody what they need to help them improve.

Joshua, MS, OT – Other professions discrediting what we bring to the table as OTs.

Kelli, MSW – The entrenchment of social injustice in this country, in particular towards women, People of Colour, immigrants, and people who live in poor areas.

Marie, MSW – Health care inequity. It is said that death is an equalizer, but it actually isn't. How people die and where they die is often dependent on affluence. The underrepresented and the underserved are not dying where they want to be. COVID is making things even harder for everyone, but people who are already at a particular threshold of poverty are even more negatively impacted. In a time when we need people around, human connection is more challenging because of COVID. Also, documentation takes away so much time from patient and family care. Being on our computers for hours is a waste of human resources. I wish it could be streamlined.

Regina, MSW – We have people suffering and I'm confused as to why we just cannot make people and their needs a high priority.

Sabine, Cultural Broker – Things are getting difficult in Portland, Maine, US, for clients. Things keep changing in a negative way. Immigrants and Blacks are the less fortunate in all this change.

Said, OTD – The Patient-Driven Payment Model (PDPM) is causing therapists to lose jobs and some graduates are having a hard time finding fieldwork placements and jobs. Patients are not getting the therapy they need as well. We are living in a world of greed. As a result of PDPM, some facilities are cutting 20–30% of their workforce in rehabilitation in the US, which is a serious concern.

Saige, Tribal Youth Engagement Manager – Just the continued racism and overall systems that are in place don't support people working collaboratively or being inclusive. One of the problems is always a concern [about] having secure funding on the State and Federal levels.

Usha, MD – Decisions made without an understanding of workflow affect the patient and providers adversely. It is very important to create foolproof systems so that we reduce the chance of communication errors and missteps in medicine. Insurance company regulations cause a lot of waste of time and energy, and delay care in some instances.

What do you see as the relationship between planetary health and human health?

Carl, PA – They are one and the same. As a species, we have removed ourselves from nature and the rest of every living thing that exists and somehow we think we are not responsible for anything that happens in the world. As my Tai Chi master says, once humans got the electric light, it was all over. The rest of the world honours the end of the day, and we do not. As long as we continue to live our lives as if we are divorced from the world around us, it's hopeless and we are a doomed species.

Islane, RN, MSN – You can't even talk about human health without talking about planetary health. We live in the environment. If you don't take care of it, I don't believe you are taking care of yourself.

Joshua, MS, OT – We treat the planet almost like we treat our bodies, these days. We only get one planet and only get one body so we should truly value them.

Kelli, MSW – When people start to become more self-aware, they come to care about themselves more and they open their eyes to see what's around them more. My hope is they will take care of what is around them a bit more. I do think there is an interconnection between emotional health and planetary health. When people are struggling to survive, it is hard to care about anything else. I also think greed makes people callous to what they are doing to the Earth.

Marie, MSW – I think it is very, very, very connected. I think the health of the planet has a direct impact on human health and wellbeing.

Patricia, BS, OT – I would like to see people of all racial and cultural backgrounds get the support needed early on in order to thrive. Education, honesty and transparency, and a true commitment to enact changes will be key to progress in the health and social care systems. Let's really look at socioeconomic disparities and provide the support and opportunities people need. I believe we can do this.

Sabine, Cultural Broker – Very connected. What happens wrong to the planet will impact human health. We need to take care of ourselves and the planet.

Said, OTD – Growing up in a developing nation let me live much closer to the land, but also in a system without the environmental protections seen in Western countries. I firmly believe there is a connection between the health of our planet and human health and we should do anything in our power to protect our planet and thereby protect humans and other living creatures.

Saige, Tribal Youth Engagement Manager – The Earth is being abused, and we feel it. I can say that relates to what we're going through at the moment (COVID-19). Earth is starting to heal itself. River rights, climate justice, and social justice, they are one and the same. Like, who's impacted most by climate change, People of Colour? It's a reality. Social justice is climate justice. The youth speak to that, so, hearing their issues and their concerns – it is one and the same.

Usha, MD – Planetary and human health are more connected than one would imagine. Just as all the organs in the human body are connected, all the systems of the planet are interdependent. We need to be cognizant of our external environment as well as our internal processes to live a conscious life.

What are your hopes and vision for health and social care systems that support the flourishing of all racial and cultural groups – clients and practitioners alike? What has inspired this vision?

Carl, PA – Our current system has to crash in order for us to create something new out of the rubble. Why don't we do the things that are obvious and need to be done? It's part of the unique dysfunction of individualism and an emphasis on being in the moment. Whether it is the current pandemic, or something else, the system has to crash the system, and then we can climb out of the rubble as Europe did after W[orld] W[ar] II. Chipping away at the edges and around the edges doesn't work. We have too many self-serving interests for people to radically change unless the change is forced upon us.

If we could work together more, then we could shift a few things by using the model we used in the interprofessional geriatric programme. We used the Turf, Team, and Town model. Turf involves helping students understand and embrace their professional roles. The Team involves building on that understanding to engage and connect with other professionals on the team. Town involves learning to serve the community as a team. If we could use that model on a macro scale, we could make a difference.

Islane, RN, MSN – My hope is to see equity in health care. When you come to the hospital, does anyone pay attention to your beliefs about health and wellness? People need to take the time to ask. My inspiration comes from my own cultural background. There are a lot of things that are taboos for a Haitian. When you don't take time to provide the right education and just prescribe medications, guess what? They won't take it. That is one simple example among many.

Joshua, MS, OT – My hope is that money doesn't become the primary object. It's the biggest barrier to having humans flourish and it inhibits us from truly caring. Money comes and goes, but people don't.

Kelli, MSW – We need universal health care – that's the first thing. It would be a joy and a complete gift. I also think interprofessional collaboration is a huge necessity. It isn't just fun to collaborate; it is a complete necessity, so people don't die. I also have a vision where hunger and homelessness are not issues here, in the wealthiest country in the world. It's completely unacceptable. I also think if children have enough to eat, and they have a safe place to live, a decent school, and parents who have time for them, we'll be raising a generation of people who have time to care about what's around them.

Marie, MSW – I think it really comes down to basic things – people need safe housing, nutritious food, access to safe transportation, and access to health care. When someone is down and out, and really disenfranchised, it manifests in their cells and in how their body manifests diseases and chronic health conditions. It's a really different playing field. My biggest wish is for social equity – this is the root of change and alleviating any unnecessary suffering. My mom was a big inspiration. She did a lot of social justice work with missions through the Catholic church. I learned a lot about people more disenfranchised than my family, and that people with the hardest lives often had a sense of joy because they had each other versus things. Also, here in the US, many people have so many resources yet are so lonely, isolated, and often lack joy or perspective. When people have each other, that impacts wellbeing. Though considered a family of humble beginnings in our community, we were close and grateful for most of what we had.

Regina, MSW – Crack the nut of racism – get at the root causes. We need to take deep dives into many systems.

Sabine, Cultural Broker – I hope to see a positive change between races – equality, where immigrants are empowered to have their voice at the table for decision-making.

Said, OTD – It benefits our clients when we do our best to see that the workforce reflects the background our clients are from. The US is the richest country in the world, but not the best in health care. We are ignoring the fact that other countries have other ways of delivering health care that is far better than us. My dream is we will do better at controlling costs, improving service delivery, and having better outcomes that will honour and support all clients, regardless of culture and race. Parts of my childhood inspire my future vision for the health and social care systems; I grew up in a country and a religion where you stand shoulder to shoulder with multiple races in your prayers and daily life. Morocco is known for its tolerance of other religions. While I am very proud to be born Moroccan, I'm equally proud to be an American, a country that has let me practise my faith as I choose and follow a professional path that lets me interact with a diverse group. There is always room for improvement, but projects like this interview are exactly what gives me hope and inspires me to have faith that health and social care systems will flourish for all.

Saige, Tribal Youth Engagement Manager – Healthcare workers' representation is important. The biggest thing is systematic changes and to be more inclusive of everyone's beliefs and traditions and letting that individual or community lead the discussion. I'm so thankful to be able to work for a tribal public health agency. A lot of the work we do is different because we know what the communities need and who we're taking direction from and are in collaboration with.

Steve, DPT – There is a huge disparity in health care. You have people who go completely bankrupt in the US because of a single health issue/event. I hope for a health care system that allows all individuals to have access to affordable quality care and medications.

Usha, MD – A health care system serving all subsets of the population appropriately needs [the] empowerment and participation of all the subsections of the population at different levels of development of the health care policy and its execution. It is much like a democracy that is represented by all the people, and not just the rich, educated, and empowered. We must remove financial incentives for any testing, surgeries, or procedures. Making sure the providers are debt-free and salaried may help attain these goals.

TABLE 11.1 Partnerships to support listening in health and social care teams: Voices of frontline workers as leaders

Listening to each other as health and social care practitioners	Questions for dialogue and connection *Each speaker decides on which question(s) they would like to answer* *(15 minutes minimum each way on selected questions)*	Journal/discussion prompts
Pride	• What are you proud of and appreciate about your profession?	1. What stood out for you among practitioner responses, peer responses, and your own responses to the interview questions?
Challenges	• What is hard, difficult, or challenging about being or becoming a practitioner in your chosen field?	
Collaboration with other practitioners	• Share about other health or social care professionals you have appreciated collaborating with.	2. Discuss what it will be like to invite other health and social care practitioners to answer the interview questions?
Listening, loving, and lifting spirits – within and across racial and cultural lines	• What have you noticed about listening, loving, and lifting spirits as a student or health or social care practitioner?	
	• What have you noticed about listening, loving, and lifting spirits within and across racial and cultural lines?	3. What action steps would you like to take to enhance the health and wellbeing of all people and all living things?
Racial and cultural identity as a practitioner	• Discuss your perspective on the role of having others (peers, therapists, colleagues, partners) listen, love, and lift your spirits in your role as a _____.	
Leadership	• Share how your racial and cultural identity has influenced you as a future practitioner.	
Giving and receiving feedback	• Discuss your experiences with collaboration and leadership.	
Concerns	• What has supported the process of giving and receiving feedback to support the best practice?	
Relationship between human and planetary health	• What concerns you most as a future health or social care practitioner?	
	• What do you see as the relationship between planetary health and human health?	
Hopes and visions (15+ minutes each way)	• What are your hopes and visions for a health care system that supports the flourishing of all racial and cultural groups – clients and practitioners alike? What has inspired this vision?	

12

TRANSFORMING EXPERIENCES IN HEALTH AND SOCIAL CARE TO IMPROVE HEALTH AND WELLBEING FOR ALL

Lives on the line: Realities of jobs in health and social care

Experiences and perspectives shared by interviewees in Chapter 11 highlight the deep love and appreciation that health and social care practitioners have for their work and also highlight their concerns. Many of these concerns pre-dated the coronavirus, yet a myriad new challenges have emerged in the pandemic. Unprecedented prioritization of the safety, health, and wellbeing of all members of the health and social care teams is a new "must".

Before the pandemic, *U.S. News & World Report* (U.S. News Staff, 2020), reported that jobs in health care dominated Best Job rankings (see Table 12.1). Higher salaries, plenty of job openings, and opportunities for promotion are characteristics used for these rankings. Many health and social care practitioners choose their profession because of a desire to help others and to experience compassion satisfaction – or feelings of self-appreciation while caring for others (Okoli et al., 2019; Smart et al., 2014; Zhang et al., 2018). They knowingly decide to accept some risk in their chosen profession (exposure to infectious diseases, violence from clients, biological hazards, etc.). However, the alarming degree of risk faced by health practitioners in the coronavirus pandemic, combined with projections of more pandemics to come as climate change unfolds, will undoubtedly change the desirability of jobs in health care until systemic changes afford all health and social care practitioners greater protection in their work.

Lack of compassion for oneself: Suicide in practitioners

Despite high levels of job satisfaction and compassion satisfaction among many health and social care practitioners, between 300 and 400 physicians kill themselves each year in the United States – double the rate of suicide in the general population

TABLE 12.1 *U.S. News & World Report 2020:* Best jobs in health care

Health care job	Best job ranking
Dentist	#1
Physician Assistant	#2
Nurse Practitioner	#4
Physician	#5
Speech-Language Pathologist	#6
Registered Nurse	#9
Physical Therapists	#10
Occupational Therapists	#17
Substance Abuse and Behavioral Disorder Counselor (could be a Social Worker)	#35
Marriage and Family Counselor (could be a Social Worker)	#51
Mental Health Counselor (could be a social worker)	#71
Clinical Social Worker	#86

Source: U.S. News Staff (2020, January 7).

and higher than rates within every other profession (Anderson, 2018). Female nurses are 12% more likely and male nurses are 40% more likely to commit suicide than women and men in the general population in the United States (Davidson et al., 2019). Some of the reasons why practitioners commit suicide include extreme job stress, the tragedies of daily work life, a sense of inadequacy, work pressures, lack of support, deep distress when mistakes are made, explicit horizontal violence in the workplace, ready access to potentially lethal drugs, mental health/substance abuse issues and "burnout" (Sinha, 2014; Walker, 2017; Wible, 2018).

Burnout

"Burnout" is described as a psychological syndrome characterized by emotional exhaustion, depersonalization, cynicism, and reduced professional efficacy (Maslach et al., 2001). Even prior to the coronavirus pandemic, burnout was rampant among health professionals in both high- and middle-to-low-income countries (Dubale et al., 2019). More than one-half of physicians, one-third of nurses, and between 69% and 78% of medical residents reported symptoms of burnout in the United States (Reith, 2018). Burnout in the coronavirus pandemic has its distinct narrative. Not only are members of health care teams (physicians, nurses, respiratory therapists, cleaning staff, etc.) threatened with contracting the virus, they are also at great risk for burnout due to overstress in an overburdened health care system (Lagasse, 2020). Lai et al. (2020) explored the mental health of frontline workers (physicians and nurses) in Chinese hospitals and found high rates of depression (50.4%), anxiety (44.6%), and insomnia (34%), with 71.5% of frontline workers reporting the psychological burden of distress in handling the many unknowns associated with the coronavirus. Correlations between burnout in health and social care practitioners and medical errors, patient mortality, dissemination of hospital-transmitted infections, decreased altruism, alcohol abuse, lower patient satisfaction, and greater job turnover are a tragic reality (Panagioti et al., 2018; Reith, 2018; Welp et al., 2015).

As we learned in Chapter 11, challenges in the workplace vary greatly among practitioners. The stress of long work hours, extreme productivity demands, time spent in documentation versus client care, and student debt are burnout factors that tend to cut across many health professions (see Table 12.2). Compassion fatigue, or the emotional toll of attempting to show compassion at all times, without time to refuel oneself, and vicarious or secondary trauma, the experiencing of trauma-related symptoms and a change in one's worldview due to exposure to client trauma, are also common burnout factors. Both can lessen job and compassion satisfaction and also result in lessening of the ability of health and social care practitioners to truly empathize with the trauma and suffering of their clients (Good Therapy, 2016; Leland & Armstrong, 2015; Peate, 2014; Smart et al., 2014). Many workplaces offer wellness, self-care, and resilience programmes as solutions to burnout in health care, yet systemic changes are necessary to improve health outcomes by improving experiences in health care for practitioners and clients alike (Stehman et al., 2019; Vogel, 2018).

Improving the experience for practitioners: From the Triple to the Quadruple Aim

In 2007, the Institute for Healthcare Improvement (IHI) created the Triple Aim, a system of linked goals that simultaneously seek to improve the patient's experience of care, lower the per capita cost, and improve the health of communities and populations (Berwick et al., 2008). It serves as an important guide for health care practitioners as they address the seemingly insurmountable problems in health care. In response to widespread burnout and compassion fatigue among health care professionals, an additional aim, the Quadruple Aim, has been proposed which seeks to improve not only the experience of care for patients but also for providers (Bodenheimer & Sinsky, 2014). The aftermath of the coronavirus pandemic calls for the adoption of the Quadruple Aim and implementation of policies to improve experiences in health and social care for practitioners and clients alike as key to improving health and wellbeing for all. Such transformation in health care requires effective leadership – both inherent leadership and designated leadership to build strong collaboration among diverse minds and hearts.

Inherent leaders: Changing lives moment by moment

Most leadership occurs in the courageous, everyday decisions and actions of ordinary people moment by moment. Practitioner experiences shared in Chapter 11 highlight that although one may not be a designated leader in a group or organization, leadership occurs by thinking about the whole, taking initiative, and moving

TABLE 12.2 Reasons for burnout among health and social care practitioners

	Social workers (Robb 2004; Smullens, 2012)	Physicians (Reith, 2018; Stehman et al., 2019)	Nurses (De Keyrel, 2018; Peters, 2018; Sherman, 2018)	Occupational therapists (Leland & Armstrong, 2015; Lyon, 2019)	Physical therapists (Jannenga, 2019; Klappa et al., 2015).
Productivity demands	Heavy caseloads and unrealistic time frames	Long work hours – average 51 hrs/week; 25% work 80 hrs/week	Stress of long work hours and continually expanding role	Productivity demands	Unrealistic productivity standards
Financial concerns and student debt	Low pay and lack of appreciation	Financial concerns	Financial stress	Student debt	Abysmal salary to debt ratio
Compassion fatigue and secondary trauma	Vicarious or secondary trauma and compassion fatigue	Second victim syndrome – trauma from adverse events	Innate desire to help others rather than self – compassion fatigue	Compassion fatigue – emotional and physical demands	Compassion fatigue
Working conditions	Adverse working conditions without foreseeable relief	Many bureaucratic tasks detract from time with patients (profits over patients)	Employer demands in the context of nurse shortages	Repetitive nature of work and lack of growth and support	Poor company cultures
Electronic Medical Record (EMR)		More time spent on Electronic Medical Record than treating patients			Cumbersome technology
Teamwork			Teamwork pressures (poor communication, conflict, and tension)		
Flexibility				Envy of more flexible careers	

individuals and groups forward in a positive direction. From the ICU nurse who lightens the mood of her colleagues as she jokes about using maxi-thin sanitary pads instead of N95 masks as personal protective equipment (PPE) to the charge nurse who organizes and leads a health team, the field of nursing identifies all nurses as leaders. As experts in human health, as educators, as caring and compassionate listeners, as advocates and role models with members of health and social care teams, and as voices for the profession – every nurse is not only an inherent leader but has the potential to become an increasingly effective leader who transforms experiences in health care (Bonsall, 2017; Thew, 2019). The same can be said for every member of the health and social care teams – social workers, intake staff, occupational therapists, physical therapists, janitors (McKenna, 2012), clients, and family members are all inherent leaders who play key roles in improving health and wellbeing for all. Case vignettes and leadership stories in previous chapters illustrate how inherent leadership in health and social care enhances the client's experience of their care and also improves the work–life experience for health and social care practitioners.

Additionally, practitioners who take courageous action when they encounter mistreatment of fellow colleagues or clients are inherent leaders who could also be called *upstanders*. *Upstander* refers to anyone who is willing to take a stand when they notice something is not right. They are guided by principles of equity, justice, respect, human dignity, freedom, and love. Despite feelings of timidity, confusion, and fear, they act on what they know to be right – they listen, they love, and they lift spirits and take whatever additional action is needed to rectify the mistreatment of others. In Chapter 5, home care nurse Robert took a courageous and principled stand when he intervened on Nahla's behalf when she was being harassed by a neighbour (vignette 5.3). Sandra, the physical therapist in Chapter 7 exhibited integrity and courage by reaching out to the resident who called their patient "fat" (vignette 7.5). Janine, in Chapter 10, courageously stood up for a CNA who was being sexually harassed by an older male client (vignette 10.3). Prevention.Action. Change (n.d.) has a website that offers a variety of resources and strategies for active bystander and upstander strategies.

Designated leaders: Building diverse teams and communities to transform health and wellbeing for humans and the planet

Listening, loving, and lifting spirits are at the heart of not only inherent leadership and upstander strategies, but also serve as a foundation for the demands of designated leadership roles. As competence, confidence, and enjoyment from leadership emerge, many upstanders and inherent leaders are either invited to take on or seek designated leadership roles where they are challenged to lead large numbers of people towards a common purpose. Those who step into designated leadership roles are called upon to build effective teams – diverse teams with strong, caring, and collaborative relationships within and across the many lines or divisions in health and social care. Although they can play a key role in meeting the Quadruple

Aim, their effectiveness is dependent on their ability to support the talents and growth of inherent leaders.

There are a variety of frameworks and conceptual guides for leadership in health care, community organizations, and the business world that apply to both inherent and designated leaders (see Table 12.3). Each call for building teams to affect both small- and large-scale change within systems, organizations, and communities. We propose the following synthesis of key elements identified in these frameworks with our model – "Leadership for transforming racial and cultural lines in health and social care" (see Table 12.4).

Leadership for transforming racial and cultural lines in health and social care

1. Modelling integrity, courage, caring, and decisive action

Both inherent and designated leaders are often called upon to lead because of their integrity, courage, caring, and ability to take principled stands and decisive action. Greta Thunberg sparked a global climate movement because of her unwavering integrity, courage, and decisive action to protect the planet and all living things. As we learned in Chapter 11, health and social care practitioners lead on multiple levels to improve lives for all people. Several of those interviewed identified and attributed their family, cultural, religious, and ethnic identities in shaping their leadership styles.

Many courageous leaders have emerged in the coronavirus pandemic. Countries with some of the most inspiring results in flattening the coronavirus curve are led by women – Prime Minister Jacinda Ardern of New Zealand, Angela Merkel, Chancellor of Germany, Prime Minister Sanna Marin of Finland, Tsai Ing-wen, President of Taiwan, Denmark's Prime Minister, Mette Frederiksen, and Iceland's Prime Minister Katrín Jakobsdóttir (Gowthaman, 2020). Each has taken swift and decisive action backed by scientific evidence, and they have also been guided by the compassion that prioritizes people over national economic interests. Their transparent and dependable communication has engendered trust among their people. Dr Anthony Fauci, director of the National Institute of Allergy and Infectious Diseases and Coronavirus Task Force adviser, is a hero to many in the United States for his honesty and no-nonsense demeanour in communicating requirements for flattening the coronavirus curve (Rosenbaum, 2020). Dr Zhong Nanshan, a pulmonologist who holds no formal office, has been China's hero in both the SARS and coronavirus pandemics for his honest warnings about the contagious nature of both viruses and for his open mourning around the loss of Dr Li Wenliang, the whistle-blowing doctor who later died of the coronavirus (Feng & Cheng, 2020). Both Dr Fauci and Dr Zhong are seen by many as reliable sources of information who demonstrate a deep love for others, the courage to speak out, and speak the truth even if it means contradicting government officials.

2. Inspiring hope, furnishing confidence, and communicating a shared vision for better health and wellbeing for all

Due to the heavy discouragement felt by many people in the world, it is essential for transformative leaders in health and social care such as Dr Fauci and Dr Zhong to persistently communicate that it is possible to achieve better health for all. Professor Sir Michael Marmot stands out as a leader who for the past 30 years has decried inequities that contribute to poor health. He is known for exposing the health–wealth gradient (see Chapter 9) and calls for evidence-based policy centred on the social determinants of health to reduce health disparities. In the report subtitled *Fair Society, Healthy Lives* (Marmot et al., 2010), Marmot and colleagues provided a vision of healthy lives in England with the enactment of the following policies:

- Give every child the best start in life.
- Enable all children, young people, and adults to maximize their capabilities and have control over their lives.
- Create fair employment and good work for all.
- Ensure a healthy standard of living for all.
- Create and develop healthy and sustainable places and communities.
- Strengthen the role and impact of ill-health prevention.

A follow-up report, *Health Equity in England: The Marmot Review 10 Years On* (Marmot et al., 2020), shows that rather than making progress, England, by not enacting these policies, has been faltering on many health indices since 2011. To some extent, Scandinavian countries have high rates of health and wellbeing because many of the policies proposed by Marmot et al. – high-quality free education and health care, ample parental leave, and a labour market model that protects against anxiety around jobs and job loss – are integrated into these societies (Lakey, 2016; Walton, 2018; World Population Review, 2020). Alleviation of poverty has been the key to making life measurably better in these nations (Matthews, 2015).

On a hopeful note, Bregman (2017) notes that rates of extreme poverty across the globe decreased from 84% in 1820 to 44% in 1981. Although these rates continued to decrease from 36% in 1990 to 10% in 2015, an average of one percentage point per year, this rate has slowed in recent years (World Bank, 2018). The coronavirus now threatens to further reverse this cherished progress by potentially pushing an extra half a billion more people into poverty (McCarthy, 2020). Implementation of a universal basic income (UBI) to mitigate the economic calamities and threats to the health, wellbeing, and livelihood of millions of people posed by the pandemic is supported by Pope Francis and many other scholars, leaders, and policymakers across the globe (Bregman, 2017; Di Santo, 2020; Santens, 2020). In fact, Spain, one of the nations hardest-hit by the pandemic, has already passed a permanent UBI (Slater, 2020). According to the United Nations, if multinational corporations, many of which reap obscene amounts of profit while evading taxes via a maze of complex loopholes – Apple, Amazon, Google, and Walmart – to

TABLE 12.3 Frameworks and conceptual guides for transformational leadership

"Collaborative leadership: Moving from top-down to team-centric" (Samur, 2019)	"What defines a true leader in health care?" (Huston, 2018)	"Leadership in interprofessional health and social care teams: A literature review" (Smith et al., 2018)	The leadership challenge (Kouzes & Posner, 2017)	Leading diverse Communities (Brown & Mazza, 2005; NCBI, 2017)	The enjoyment of leadership (Jackins, 1987)
Tap into collective intelligence	Envision a desired future – an optimal working environment	Overall leader is necessary – Facilitate shared leadership	Model the way – reflect shared values and achieve small wins	Building hopeful environments to welcome diversity – every person and every issue counts	Think about the group as a whole – Elicit the thinking of the group
Clarify a common purpose – all employees as caregivers	Foster innovation and change with open communication and collaboration	Support transformation and change	Inspire a shared vision – uplifting, exciting, and meaningful	Healing ourselves to change the world – venting for clearer thinking	Inspire, lead, and organize
Keep communication open – appreciating others and purposeful conversations	Build effective teams with a shared vision – empower full potential of team members	Personal qualities – enthusiasm, commitment, empathy, knowledge of people	Challenge the process – search for opportunities for growth and take risks	Becoming effective allies – one-to-one relationships are key to break mistrust and build coalitions across group lines	Model integrity, courage, commitment to group goals, and decisive action
Build partnership skills – all experiences are valid	Create a positive work culture – model honesty and integrity; admit and take ownership of mistakes	Goal alignment with clear and inspiring vision	Enabling others to act – foster collaboration and delegate power	Empowering leaders to lead – training leadership teams	Listening to promote healing and fresh thinking

Don't waste time – build efficient integration into workflows	Expose all members of health teams to leadership training	Creativity and innovation – balance harmony and debate	Encourage the heart – recognize contributions, celebrate team accomplishments	Importance of individual initiative	Creating and following policies
Don't be afraid to show vulnerability and ask for help		Sustain clear communication and team building		Changing hearts through stories	Value of individual leadership – problems with co-leadership
		Leadership clarity and direction setting		Integrity to take principled stands	Handling attacks and growth as a leader
		External liaison – represents the team to develop resources		Ongoing support for leaders and handling attacks	Produce other leaders
		Ensure skill mix and diversity		Leaders change more from generosity than criticism	Enjoyment and satisfaction in leadership
		Clinical and contextual expertise		Trusted leaders admit and correct mistakes	

TABLE 12.4 Leadership for transforming cultural and racial lines in health and social care

Model components
1. Modelling integrity, courage, caring, and decisive action
2. Inspiring hope, furnishing confidence, and communicating a shared vision for better health and wellbeing for all
3. Eliciting the thinking of the group to liberate creative ideas and develop best policies and practices
4. Committing to group goals, policies, and practices
5. Promoting listening exchanges to facilitate healing and unity within and across racial and cultural lines
6. Supporting appreciations of all health and social care team members, including oneself, and the planet
7. Collaborating to develop and implement action steps that lift spirits
8. Inviting constructive feedback to optimize collaborative efforts
9. Infusing enjoyment and playfulness in collaborative endeavours

name just a few, were fairly taxed, a modest UBI could be funded and distributed in countries across the globe (Wignaraja & Horvath, 2020). In addition to visions for a UBI, proposals for permaculture (Permaculture Research Institute, 2020), circular economies (Laita, 2019), worker cooperatives (Anzilotti, 2018), and a global Green New Deal (Corbett, 2020), each centred on sustaining all life, invite humanity towards a brighter and healthier future.

Practitioners in Chapter 11 echo the hopes and visions of Marmot and others for health and social care systems that support the flourishing of all racial and cultural groups – clients and practitioners alike. Achieving equity in health care, eliminating anti-Black racism and all forms of oppression, increasing diversity among health and social care practitioners, and creating systemic changes in health and social care that replace profit-driven models with models that prioritize love and caring for humans and the planet are underscored.

3. Eliciting the thinking of groups to liberate creative ideas and develop best policies and practices

As Kouzes and Posner (2017) noted, a leader must "Listen, and listen, and listen some more" (p. 218). Eliciting the voices of health and social care practitioners, modelled in Chapter 11, is an example of liberating the ideas of others to create better health and social care. An effective leader cannot think for multiracial and multicultural groups but supporting listening among health and social care team members can unleash creative thinking within these diverse groups. Collaborative goals and effective policies and practices can be developed and problems, both large and small, can be solved. The following practices are recommended to elicit thinking within racially and culturally diverse groups:

- Opening Circles – starting meetings with the sharing of news and goods or highs and lows is a good way to build connections, energize a group, and free up thinking (Bridges Coaching, 2019).
- Listening to All Perspectives – giving every group member a chance to speak once before anyone speaks twice on a particular issue liberates the broadest thinking possible (Shafaki, 2018).
- Think and Listens – giving group members equal time to think aloud about a topic or problem, either in pairs or small groups, while listeners refrain from commenting or judging the content of what is shared liberates creative thinking (Shafaki, 2018).
- Listening Exchanges/Partnerships – creating confidential opportunities for team members to connect and vent frustration, tension, and grief with each other enhances flexible thinking (Jackins, 1987).

4. *Committing to group goals, policies, and practices*

The World Health Organization (WHO) is committed to the goal of health for all, and health and social care practitioners are committed to the goal of enhancing the health and wellbeing of their clients, communities, and populations. Policies and practices support the achievement of goals, yet the word "policy", in particular, can have negative connotations because of the many overbearing rules we all experienced in our lives as young people. In fact, both individuals and groups need policies as guides for actions in life and perhaps this has never been so clear as within the coronavirus pandemic – wash your hands frequently, maintain physical distancing, wear a face mask, treat each other and yourself well, clean up after yourself, listen without interrupting, show up on time, seek support for oneself, take a 1-minute break and rest your eyes from teleconferencing every 30 minutes, etc. On a broader scale, the transformation of racial and cultural lines in health care is occurring because of commitment to collaborative goals and effective policies and practices such as those identified by the World Health Organization (WHO, 2013), TeamSTEPPS (Agency for Healthcare Research and Quality, 2020), Healthy People 2020 (Office of Disease Prevention and Health Promotion, 2020), and hundreds of other health and social care agencies.

Some practitioners in Chapter 11 called for elevating the voices of Black, Indigenous, and People of Colour or People of the Global Majority in health and social care. Only then can collaborative goals and policies be developed, and collaborative action taken towards the achievement of health and wellbeing for all people. Several policies and practices that leaders can implement so that multiracial and multicultural groups have a voice in the transformation of health and social care include:

- Supporting the leadership of underrepresented racial and cultural groups.
- Using speaking order by inviting oppressed groups to speak before dominant groups (i.e. young people before older people, Black, Indigenous, People of

Colour or People of the Global Majority before white people, females before males, etc.) reverses the dynamics of oppression and creates the safety for marginalized people to reclaim their essential and powerful voices. Inclusive group goals can be developed.

- Using effective translators in individual and group meetings.
- Incorporating a restorative minute of silence in meetings after every 20–30 minutes to allow translators and those who do not speak the dominant language some mental rest.
- Making environments accessible and welcoming to people of all backgrounds and abilities.
- Honouring Indigenous people by acknowledging occupancy on their lands.
- Offering basic and advanced racial and cultural awareness and action training to health and social care providers that can focus on:
  - inviting clients to share important racial and cultural values and beliefs
  - responding to those values and beliefs in a culturally responsive manner
  - taking action against anti-Black racism and other forms of oppression
  - support in recovery from mistakes while dismantling anti-Black racism and other forms of oppression
  - opportunities for ongoing healing from the effects of oppression and internali zed oppression within and across racial and cultural lines.

5. Promoting listening exchanges to facilitate healing and unity within and across all racial and cultural lines

We transform ourselves inwardly by offering our listening and by inviting others to listen to us. We mutually heal, and the world transforms. Each practitioner in Chapter 11 underscored the significance of listening in their work. Several practitioners noted that it is important to take care of their own emotional health and wellbeing in order to be available to their clients. They highlighted the value of being listened to by friends, family members, or professionals. Others suggested that if listening to each other was a regular occurrence, practitioners would be in much better shape to handle the challenges before them – a little resource goes a long way. When practitioners are listened to with compassion, there is a trickle-down effect and their clients benefit.

Hence, readers who have experienced the restorative and healing benefits of listening partnerships or listening exchanges may want to teach the skills of listening, loving, and lifting spirits to both clients and colleagues in order to accelerate a positive transformation in health and social care. More than ever, humans across all walks of life are in need of places to show themselves more fully to each other as they release collective grief and fear as our species struggles to heal from the vast losses associated with climate change, a collapsing society and poverty, ongoing wars, and multiple epidemics and pandemics. As we heal together, we will generate creative, life-affirming solutions to the myriad problems we face in health and social care.

Confidential venting with trusted peers has been widely recognized as an important element of recovery for people with mental health challenges for a number of years, and is now being effectively utilized in disease management and prevention and perinatal care when using a trauma-informed, culturally responsive lens (Group Peer Support [GPS], 2020). Studies also show that thoughtfully provided peer support enables health and social care practitioners to actively process relationships with clients and recover from highly stressful situations – especially when non-judgmental listening is provided and confidentiality is assured (O'Connell, 2016; Roberts, 2012; van Pelt, 2008; van Roy et al., 2015). Common concerns about the stigma associated with seeking help and showing emotions tend to be bypassed when peers, as equals, are reminded that releasing and processing our feelings by talking, shedding a few angry words or tears, or laughing with someone we feel connected to is a natural process. This process contributes to our emotional health and wellbeing and allows us to think more clearly about ourselves and those around us. Letting people know they may derive equal or even greater satisfaction in the listener role compared to being listened to, because they can learn to be a vital support for other peers, may increase interest.

Teaching the skills of listening, loving, and lifting spirits often works best by starting with one individual and then building towards a small group as the leader's skill and confidence develop. Given the nature of historical trauma, oppression, and the stresses that are particular to racial, cultural, and occupational groups, gathering people from similar identity groups may initially be necessary to ensure safety for racial and cultural emotional exchanges to occur. For example, Black people, Indigenous people, other People of Colour, white people, women, men, people with disabilities, doctors, nurses, etc. may find it very helpful to meet with just members of their own racial or cultural group to address their specific concerns and experiences. Yet on the other hand, sometimes including trusted allies from other groups may be the key to creating a safe environment for open and loving exchanges. A key role for the leader is to initiate and sustain listening partnership groups to contradict the discouragement that leads people to isolate themselves. Additionally, always enlisting at least one key support person who can offer their support, love, and appreciation enables teachers and leaders to promote listening and healing within and across racial and cultural lines more effectively.

6.   Supporting appreciations of health and social care team members, including oneself, and the planet

In Chapter 11, several practitioners shared that they are well aware their co-workers benefit from being appreciated for their important and often difficult work. One practitioner carries around a stack of appreciation cards and hands them out to her colleagues to lift their spirits. Another practitioner shares appreciations of her co-workers with their supervisors. Crowds around the world shout, cheer, clap, bang on pots, howl, and break into song to show solidarity and deep appreciation for frontline workers and community heroes in the coronavirus pandemic – nurses, first responders, doctors, and grocery store workers. The many workers behind the scenes who also kept and continue to keep us alive – respiratory therapists, janitors and housekeepers, intake staff, retail workers, farmers, delivery truck drivers, technology workers, and other health practitioners to name a few, also deserve our highest regard. Love, caring, and appreciation in its many forms (recognition, emotional support, good working conditions, affordable health care, and living wages) is vital fuel for all workers. The following examples highlight "shout outs" in support of a few of the many health and social care practitioners who deserve recognition.

Nurses and doctors

Nurses are the largest segment of the health care workforce (WHO, 2017) and the most trusted profession (National Nurses United, 2020). In recognition of the significant work of both nurses, for promoting health and saving lives, and of midwives, whose minds, hearts, and hands guide precious new babies and their mothers along the often perilous birthing journey, WHO declared 2020 the Year of the Nurse and Midwife (WHO, 2019). In further appreciation of nurses, health care leaders are developing policies and practices to better prepare, protect, and support nurses in their essential role in pandemics and other health crises (Mason & Friese, 2020), and to stop the devastating effects of lateral violence among nurses (Castronovo et al., 2016). In appreciation of each other for their hard work and dedication to saving lives and improving health, physicians are offering support to one another. Wible (2019) and her colleagues have developed programmes to reduce physician suicide rates, and hundreds of psychiatrists are volunteering their time on helplines that offer free support to physicians experiencing an emotional crisis in the pandemic (Cheney, 2020).

Occupational and physical therapists

Occupational therapists make profound contributions towards enhancing health and wellness for all people, especially for people with disabilities. They support participation in everyday activities that people want, need, and love to do. In recognition of their essential role, occupational therapists are being welcomed in remote parts of the world where fuller participation in everyday activities has been but a dream for many people with disabilities (Occupational Therapists Without Borders, n.d.). Physical therapists have an extraordinary ability to support all people in moving more freely with less pain, more strength, more independence, more flexibility, more endurance, and more joy in living. Increasing awareness of the vital role that physical therapists play is compelling lawmakers in the U.S. House of Representatives to introduce the Physical Therapist Workforce and Patient Access Act that addresses the critical shortage of physical therapists and physical therapy professionals, particularly in rural areas (Overman, 2019).

Social workers and physician assistants

Social workers transform the lives of individuals, families, and communities by bringing a social justice lens, heartfelt listening, and connections to vital resources in their work with people who are disenfranchised and disempowered. Using a strengths-based approach to empower oppressed people, a social worker's positive impact on communities is being increasingly noted (Truell, 2018). Appreciation for social workers has fuelled social work to become one of the fastest-growing professions internationally (Truell, 2018). Physician assistants also play a vital role in supporting health and saving lives. They are a key solution to the critical shortage of physicians, resulting in physician assistants becoming one of the most sought-after health professionals (Wu, 2018).

Health and social care practitioners and the Earth

Fortunately, a deep love and appreciation for Earth, our life-sustaining planet, and an increasing awareness of the interconnection between human and planetary health are fuelling climate activism among many members of the health and social care teams (Kreslake et al., 2018). Meaningful support and appreciation of all health and social care team members globally and locally, including oneself and the living Earth, can seem daunting. Yet it is actually enjoyable and absolutely possible – especially in collaborative partnerships grounded in the reality that every contribution towards human and planetary health and wellbeing matters. Since many health and social care practitioners tend to think well about others, often to the detriment of their own wellbeing, supporting self-care and self-love for the practitioner is paramount. In reality, we cannot be fully effective allies to our clients, nor have a depth of attention for the current climate crisis, if we do not support appreciation and caring for ourselves, each other, our work, and the beautiful, nurturing world around us.

7. Collaborating to develop and implement action steps to lift spirits

Most practitioners in Chapter 11 highlighted tremendous satisfaction in collaborating with others to improve their clients' health and wellbeing. Physician Raj Panjabi demonstrates collaboration on a large scale. He works with a variety of practitioners and community partners to "bring health care to everyone, everywhere." In response to the limited access to health care for hundreds of millions of people living in rural areas across the globe, he and his team formed the non-profit organization, Last Mile Health, to train community health workers with 30 essential life-saving skills (combatting infectious diseases, supporting family planning and maternal/neonatal health, first aid, HIV/AIDS treatment, etc.) that can potentially save the lives of 30 million people by 2030 (Panjabi, 2017). Community health workers are projected to play an ever-more significant role in addressing health and wellbeing in the 21st century (Housekeeper, 2019).

Effective leaders support collaborative action by fostering inherent leadership and artfully managing inevitable conflict that arises in groups using the team skills identified in Chapter 7. Inviting joint participation and delegating responsibilities are also essential in order to accomplish decisive and meaningful progress in health and social care.

8. Inviting constructive feedback to optimize collaborative efforts

Always keeping an eye towards the improvement of our endeavours, leaders need a balance of appreciation and constructive feedback. Many of the practitioners in Chapter 11 stated that they welcome constructive criticism, particularly when it is offered immediately, to provide optimal care. Brown and Mazza (2005) describe a feedback process for leaders called "self-estimation". This supportive process involves gathering a group of key constituents to provide leaders with both positive feedback and constructive feedback in a manner that not only enables leaders to grow and change, but also develops a shared sense of community for all participants. Self-estimation includes the following steps:

- identifying a group facilitator
- asking a leader to identify key constituents who can provide them with feedback on both their strengths and areas for improvement
- gathering the key constituents and establishing confidentiality
- inviting all participants, including the leader, to participate in listening partnerships to clarify what they see as the leader's strengths and areas for improvement
- inviting the leader to first share their own perceptions of their strengths and areas for improvement
- inviting constituents to then provide feedback on any additional strengths and areas for improvement they have noted
- asking constituents how they can help the leader improve their leadership.

9. Infusing enjoyment and playfulness in collaborative endeavours

Recognizing the epidemic of burnout in health care even prior to the coronavirus pandemic, the Institute for Healthcare Improvement (IHI) developed a "Framework for Improving Joy at Work" as a "step toward creating safe, humane places for people to find meaning and purpose in their work" (Perlo et al., 2017. p 8). Four recommended steps for leaders include:

1. Ask the staff, "What matters to you?"
2. Identify unique impediments to joy in work in the local context.
3. Commit to a systems approach to making joy in work a shared responsibility at all levels of the organization.

4. Use improvement science to test approaches to improving joy in work in your organization.

Perlo et al., 2017, p. 8

These four steps do not ignore systemic barriers to joy in the workplace such as workload, staffing, and the Electronic Health Record, but empower health and social care teams to ask important questions of one another, collaboratively identify winnable victories, and take action together to improve daily work life.

The IHI also identifies the importance of addressing fairness and equity to create joy in the workplace. Similarly, in response to reports that various racial and ethnic groups experience less joy at work, the National Health Service (NHS) in England explored this phenomenon and found significant disparities between the experiences of white employees and the experiences of Black, minority, and ethnic employees. They also found that sites with the highest rates of discrimination against minorities had the lowest patient experience scores (Dawson, 2009). Ten years later, the experience of discrimination against ethnic minority staff and patients continues to be a health service failure (Kmietowicz et al., 2019). Not surprisingly, in Chapter 11, several practitioners identified systems of oppression and lack of awareness of different racial and cultural groups in oneself, colleagues, and clients as key challenges in their work.

Not surprisingly, the relationship between increasing diversity in the workplace and improving not only productivity, creativity, and innovation, but also workplace happiness is also being increasingly cited (Hall, 2019; Pelletier, 2017). The Henry Ford Health System, a champion of health care equity, administered a Gallup Employee Engagement survey and found that employees participating in health care equity work were seven times more engaged than other employees (Perlo et al., 2017). The IHI document, "Achieving Health Equity: A Guide for Health Care Organizations", offers an important framework that a health care leader can use to improve health equity for their staff and the communities they serve (Wyatt et al., 2016).

Conclusion

Whether one functions as an inherent or designated leader, transforming racial and cultural lines in health and social care by building connections within teams is a joyous and rewarding activity. It is our birthright as humans to be leaders in creating a just, caring, and sustainable world for all people and all living things. As we exchange listening, loving, and lifting spirits with people within and across racial and cultural lines, we are engaged in a revolutionary act. We change our own lives, the lives of all people and the world around us. It is our destiny as members of health and social care teams to unite with each other in our inherent caring, our potential for limitless creative thinking, and our desire for joyful and tear-filled collaborative action to support health and wellbeing for all. Table 12.5 invites listening partners to explore inherent and designated leadership experiences in their own

TABLE 12.5 Partnerships to embolden leadership

Engaged listening to embolden leadership 1	*Questions for dialogue and connection* *Each speaker decides on which question(s) they would like to answer* *(15 minutes minimum each way on selected questions)*	*Journal/discussion prompts*
Leaders in your life **Your leadership**	• Discuss the traits you have admired in both inherent and designated leaders. • What specifically have you learned from leaders of different racial and cultural backgrounds that has affected your leadership? • Discuss examples of leadership within your family. • Discuss your experiences as an inherent leader and as a designated leader, and whether you had to overcome feelings of fear, inadequacy, or reluctance to lead. • Discuss your leadership or backing of leaders of diverse groups. • What strengths do you bring to leadership roles and what challenges have you experienced? • What are you most proud of as a leader? • Discuss the support you have experienced or the lack thereof as a leader. • Discuss your awareness of when it makes sense to lead and when it makes sense to follow.	1. Identify goals for yourself as both an inherent and designated leader. 2. What feelings do you need to overcome to take bold action? 3. Share your experiences in making mistakes as a leader, what you learned, and how you have grown. 4. Discuss times when you have effectively decided to follow rather than to lead.

lives and to recognize the leadership of racially and culturally diverse individuals. They are asked to identify leadership goals to help them take bold action towards eliminating racial and cultural disparities in health and wellbeing.

References

Agency for Healthcare Research and Quality (2020, January). *Pocket Guide: TeamSTEPPS.* www.ahrq.gov/teamstepps/instructor/essentials/pocketguide.html

Anderson, P. (2018, May 7). Physicians experience highest suicide rate of any profession. Medscape. www.medscape.com/viewarticle/896257

Anzilotti, E. (2018, May 21). More U.S. businesses are becoming worker co-ops: Here's why? Fast Company. www.fastcompany.com/40572926/more-u-s-businesses-are-becoming-worker-co-ops-heres-why

Berwick, D. M., Nolan, T. W., & Whittington, J. (2008). The Triple Aim: Care, health, and cost. *Health Affairs, 27*(3), 759–769. https://doi.org/10.1377/hlthaff.27.3.759

Bodenheimer, T., & Sinsky, C. (2014). From Triple to Quadruple Aim: Care of the patient requires care of the provider. *The Annals of Family Medicine, 12*(6), 573–576. https://doi.org/10.1370/afm.1713

Bonsall, L. (2017, February 10). All nurses are leaders. NursingCenter. Blog post. www.nursingcenter.com/ncblog/february-2017/all-nurses-are-leaders

Bregman, R. (2017). *Utopia for realists: And how we can get there.* New York: Bloomsbury Publishing.

Bridges Coaching (2019, March 24). Three compelling reasons to kickstart any conversation or meeting with the high/low question. Blog post. www.bridgescoaching.net/blog/3-compelling-reasons-to-kickstart-any-conversation-or-meeting-with-the-high-low-question

Brown, C. R., & Mazza, G. J. (2005). *Leading diverse communities: A how to guide from healing to action* (Revised ed.). San Francisco, CA: Jossey-Bass.

Castronovo, M. A., Pullizzi, A., & Evans, S. (2016). Nurse bullying: A review and a proposed solution. *Nursing Outlook, 64*(3), 208–214. https://doi.org/10.1016/j.outlook.2015.11.008

Cheney, C. (2020, April 24). Coronavirus: Help line launched to support mental health of physicians. HealthLeaders. www.healthleadersmedia.com/clinical-care/coronavirus-help-line-launched-support-mental-health-physicians

Corbett, J. (2020, March 19). Global Green New Deal supporters urge world leaders to learn from coronavirus to tackle climate crisis. Common Dreams. www.commondreams.org/news/2020/03/18/global-green-new-deal-supporters-urge-world-leaders-learn-coronavirus-tackle-climate

Davidson, J. E., Proudfoot, J., Lee, K., & Zisook, S. (2019). Nurse suicide in the United States: Analysis of the Center for Disease Control 2014 national violent death reporting system dataset. *Archives of Psychiatric Nursing, 33*(5), 16–21. https://doi.org/10.1016/j.apnu.2019.04.006

Dawson, J. (2009, July). *Does the experience of staff working in the NHS link to the patient experience of care?* Aston Business School. https://assets.publishing.service.gov.uk/government/uploads/system/uploads/attachment_data/file/215457/dh_129662.pdf

De Keyrel, A. (2018, June 13). The biggest causes of nurse burnout and what you can do. MED+ED: web solutions. www.mededwebs.com/blog/well-being-index/the-biggest-causes-of-nurse-burnout-and-what-you-can-do

Di Santo, D. (2020, April 18). Pope Francis calls for a universal basic income. *The Trumpet.* www.thetrumpet.com/22233-pope-francis-calls-for-universal-basic-income

Dubale, B. W., Friedman, L. E., Chemali, Z., Denninger, J. W., Mehta, D. H., Alem, A., … Gelaye, B. (2019). Systematic review of burnout among healthcare providers in sub-Saharan Africa. *BMC Public Health, 19,* 1247. https://doi.org/10.1186/s12889-019-7566-7

Feng, E., & Cheng, A. (2020, April, 2). They call him a hero: Dr. Zhong is the public face of China's war against the coronavirus. NPR: Goats and Soda: Stories of Life in a Changing World. www.npr.org/sections/goatsandsoda/2020/04/02/825957192/dr-zhong-is-the-supreme-commander-in-china-s-war-against-coronavirus

Good Therapy (2016, July 14). Vicarious trauma. GoodTherapy. Blog post. www.goodtherapy.org/blog/psychpedia/vicarious-trauma

Gowthaman, N. (2020, April 17). Coronavirus: How have women-led countries flattened the curve? HERSTORY. https://yourstory.com/herstory/2020/04/coronavirus-women-led-countries-flattened-curve

GPS (2020). Group Peer Support. https://grouppeersupport.org/

Hall, A. (2019, June 27). 7 reasons diversity and inclusion is vital to your success. The Olson Group. https://theolsongroup.com/diversity-and-inclusion-vital-to-succcess/

Housekeeper, E. (2019, April 30). 5 of the fastest-growing public health careers. UVM OutReach. https://learn.uvm.edu/blog/blog-health/public-health-job-outlook

Huston, C. J. (2018, September). What defines a true leader in healthcare? *Today's Wound Clinic, 12*(9). www.todayswoundclinic.com/articles/what-defines-true-leader-healthcare

Jackins, H. (1987). *The enjoyment of leadership.* Seattle, WA: Rational Island Publishers.

Jannenga, H. (2019, July 29). Best of 2019: Burning and churning: Why PTs are leaving patient care. Evidence in Motion. www.evidenceinmotion.com/blog/2019/07/29/health-care-burnout-solving-the-problem/

Klappa, S. G., Fulton, L. E., Cerier, L., Peña, A., Sibenaller, A., & Klappa, S. P. (2015). Compassion fatigue among physiotherapists and physical therapists around the world. *Global Journal of Medical, Physical and Health Education, 3,* 124–137.

Kmietowicz, Z., Ladher, N., Rao, M., Salway, S., Abbasi, K., & Adebowale, V. (2019). Ethnic minority staff and patients: A health service failure. *British Medical Journal, 365,* l2226. https://doi.org/10.1136/bmj.l2226

Kouzes, J., & Posner, B. Z. (2017). *The leadership challenge: How to make extraordinary things happen in an organization.* Hoboken, NJ: John Wiley & Sons, Inc.

Kreslake, J. M., Sarfaty, M., Roser-Renouf, C., Leiserowitz, A. A., & Maibach, E. W. (2018). The critical roles of health professionals in climate change prevention and preparedness. *American Journal of Public Health, 108*(Suppl._2), S68–S69. https://doi.org/10.2105/ajph.2017.304044

Lagasse, J. (2020, March 16). Healthcare workers risk burnout, exposure in wake of coronavirus pandemic. HEALTHCARE FINANCE. www.healthcarefinancenews.com/news/healthcare-workers-risk-burnout-exposure-wake-coronavirus-pandemic

Lai, J., Ma, S., Wang, Y., Cai, Z., Hu, J., Wei, N., … Hu, S. (2020). Factors associated with mental health outcomes among health care workers exposed to Coronavirus disease 2019. *JAMA Network Open, 3*(3), e203976. https://doi:10.1001/jamanetwork open.2020.3976

Laita, S. (2019, March 13). The updated Finnish road map to a circular economy offers a new foundation for funding well-being. SITRA. www.sitra.fi/en/news/updated-finnish-road-map-circular-economy-offers-new-foundation-funding-well/

Lakey, G. (2016). *Viking economics: How the Scandinavians got it right – and how we can, too.* Brooklyn, NY: Melville House.

Leland, N. E., & Armstrong, M. (2015). Compassion fatigue: A scoping review of the literature. *American Journal of Occupational Therapy, 69*(Suppl._1), 6911505109p1. https://doi.org/10.5014/ajot.2015.69s1-rp207c

Lyon, S. (2019, January 20). Occupational therapy and burnout: What it is and how to fix it. OTPotential. https://otpotential.com/blog/occupational-therapy-burnout

Marmot, M., Allen, J., Boyce, T., Goldblatt, P., & Morrison, J. (2020). *Health equity in England: The Marmot Review 10 years on.* London: Institute of Health Equity.

Marmot, M., Allen, J., Goldblatt, P., Boyce, T., McNeish, D., Grady, M., & Geddes, I. (2010). *The Marmot Review: Fair society, healthy lives.* London: UCL.

Maslach, C., Schaufeli, W. B., & Leiter, M. P. (2001). Job burnout. *Annual Review of Psychology, 52*(1), 397–422. https://doi.org/10.1146/annurev.psych.52.1.397

Mason, D. J., & Friese, C. R. (2020, March 19). Protecting health care workers against COVID-19: And being prepared for future pandemics. JAMA Health Forum. https://jamanetwork.com/channels/health-forum/fullarticle/2763478

Matthews, D. (2015, November 11). Denmark, Finland, and Sweden are proof that poverty in the US doesn't have to be this high. Vox. www.vox.com/policy-and-politics/2015/11/11/9707528/finland-poverty-united-states

McCarthy, N. (2020, April 12). The coronavirus pandemic could push half a billion people into poverty. World Economic Forum. www.weforum.org/agenda/2020/04/coronavirus-pandemic-half-a-billion-people-into-poverty/

McKenna, M. (2012, September 1). Clean sweep: Hospitals bring janitors to the front lines of infection control. *Scientific American.* www.scientificamerican.com/article/hospitals-bring-janitors-front-lines-of-infection-control/

National Coalition Building Institute (2017). About NCBI. https://ncbi.org/about-us/

National Nurses United (2020, January 6). Nurses top Gallup poll as most trusted profession for 18th consecutive year. Press release. www.nationalnursesunited.org/press/nurses-top-gallup-poll-most-trusted-profession-18th-consecutive-year

O'Connell, L. A. (2016, March–April). Support group gives nurses a chance to process feelings. National Association of Catholic Chaplains. www.nacc.org/vision/2016-mar-apr/support-group-gives-nurses-a-chance-to-process-feelings-by-lisa-a-oconnell/

Occupational Therapists Without Borders (n.d). Collaborate – learn – grow – make a difference. http://otwithoutborders.com/

Office of Disease Prevention and Health Promotion (2020). How legal and policy levers can amplify efforts to reach healthy people goals. HealthyPeople.gov www.healthypeople.gov/2020/law-and-health-policy/topic/policy-levers

Okoli, C. T. C., Seng, S., Otachi, J. K., Higgins, J. T., Lawrence, J., Lykins, A., & Bryant, E. (2019). A cross-sectional examination of factors associated with compassion satisfaction and compassion fatigue across healthcare workers in an academic medical centre. *International Journal of Mental Health Nursing.* https://doi.org/10.1111/inm.12682

Overman, D. (2019, May 19). House of reps takes on physical therapist shortage. Physical Therapy Products. www.ptproductsonline.com/practice-management/staffing/house-reps-takes-physical-therapist-shortage/

Panagioti, M., Geraghty, K., Johnson, J., Zhou, A., Panagopoulou, E., Chew-Graham, C., … Esmail, A. (2018). Association between physician burnout and patient safety, professionalism, and patient satisfaction: A systematic review and meta-analysis. *Journal of the American Medical Association: Internal Medicine, 178*(10), 1317–1331. https://doi.org/10.1001/jamainternmed.2018.3713

Panjabi, R. (2017). *No one should die because they live too far from a doctor.* [Video file].www.ted.com/talks/raj_panjabi_no_one_should_die_because_they_live_too_far_from_a_doctor/transcript

Peate, I. (2014). Compassion fatigue: The toll of emotional labour. *British Journal of Nursing*, *23*(5), 251. https://doi:10.12968/bjon.2014.23.5.251

Pelletier, P. (2017, March 11). Workplace happiness: Using diversity to create community. Gulf Business. https://gulfbusiness.com/workplace-happiness-using-diversity-create-community/

Perlo J., Balik, B., Swensen, S., Kabcenell, A., Landsman, J., & Feeley, D. (2017). *IHI Framework for Improving Joy in Work*. IHI White Paper. Cambridge, MA: Institute for Healthcare Improvement. www.ihi.org/resources/Pages/IHIWhitePapers/Framework-Improving-Joy-in-Work.aspx

Permaculture Research Institute (2020). What is permaculture? www.permaculturenews.org/what-is-permaculture/

Peters, E. (2018, October). Compassion fatigue in nursing: A concept analysis. *Nursing Forum*, *53*(4), 466–480. https://doi.org/10.1111/nuf.12274

Prevention.Action.Change (n.d.) Bystander and upstander strategies. Handout. https://documentcloud.adobe.com/link/track?uri=urn%3Aaaid%3Ascds%3AUS%3A1b7fc481-0633-44f2-a9e5-ef47c1443686

Reith, T. P. (2018). Burnout in United States healthcare professionals: A narrative review. *Cureus, 10*(12), e3681. https://doi.org/10.7759/cureus.3681

Robb, M. (2004). Burned out – and at risk. NASW Insurance Trust. https://naswassurance.org/pdf/PP_Burnout_Final.pdf

Roberts, M. (2012, March). Balint groups: A tool for personal and professional resilience. *Canadian Family Physician, 58*(3), 245. www.ncbi.nlm.nih.gov/pmc/articles/PMC3303639/

Rosenbaum, R. (2020, March 23). How Cornell's Dr. Anthony Fauci became America's most trusted disease expert. *The Cornell Daily Sun*. https://cornellsun.com/2020/03/23/how-dr-anthony-fauci-m-d-66-became-americas-most-trusted-disease-expert/

Samur, A. (2019, March 19). Collaborative leadership: Moving from top-down to team-centric. Slack. Blog post. https://slackhq.com/collaborative-leadership-top-down-team-centric

Santens, S. (2020, April 8). The future of the United States depends on the immediate adoption of UBI. Gerald Huff: Fund for Humanity. https://fundforhumanity.org/learn-about-universal-basic-income-and-the-future-of-the-united-states/

Shafaki, A. (2018). Productive meetings. Born Trainer. www.borntrainer.com/workshops/productive-meetings

Sherman, R. O. (2018, March 1). The impact of financial stress on performance. Emerging RN Leader. www.emergingrnleader.com/impact-financial-stress-performance/

Sinha, P. (2014, September 4). Opinion: Why do doctors commit suicide? The New York Times. www.nytimes.com/2014/09/05/opinion/why-do-doctors-commit-suicide.html

Slater, N. (2020, April 8). Spain's UBI is a wake-up call for Americans. Current Affairs. www.currentaffairs.org/2020/04/spains-ubi-is-a-wake-up-call-for-americans

Smart, D., English, A., James, J., Wilson, M., Daratha, K. B., Childers, B., & Magera, C. (2014). Compassion fatigue and satisfaction: A cross-sectional survey among US healthcare workers. *Nursing & Health Sciences, 16*(1), 3–10. https://doi.org/10.1111/nhs.12068

Smith, T., Fowler-Davis, S., Nancarrow, S., Ariss, S. M. B., & Enderby, P. (2018). Leadership in interprofessional health and social care teams: A literature review. *Leadership in Health Services, 31*(4), 452–467. https://doi.org/10.1108/lhs-06-2016-0026

Smullens, S. K. (2012, Fall). What I wish I had known: Burnout and self-care in our social work profession. *The New Social Worker*. www.socialworker.com/feature-articles/field-placement/What_I_Wish_I_Had_Known_Burnout_and_Self-Care_in_Our_Social_Work_Profession/

Stehman, C. R., Testo, Z., Gershaw, R. S., & Kellogg, A. R. (2019). Burnout, drop out, suicide: Physician loss in emergency medicine, part I. *Western Journal of Emergency Medicine*, *20*(3), 485. www.ncbi.nlm.nih.gov/pmc/articles/PMC6526882/pdf/wjem-20–485.pdf

Thew, J. (2019, June 28). Hone nurse listening skills for a better patient experience. HealthLeaders. www.healthleadersmedia.com/nursing/hone-nurse-listening-skills-better-patient-experience

Truell, R. (2018, July 2). Social work is booming worldwide – because it's proven to work. *The Guardian*. www.theguardian.com/society/2018/jul/02/social-work-booming-worldwide-costa-rica

U.S. News Staff (2020, January 7). How the U.S. news ranks the best jobs. *U.S. News & World Report: Money*. https://money.usnews.com/money/careers/articles/how-us-news-ranks-the-best-jobs

van Pelt, F. (2008). Peer support: Healthcare professionals supporting each other after adverse medical events. *Quality & Safety in Health Care*, *17*(4), 249. doi: 10.1136/qshc.2007.025536

Van Roy, K., Vanheule, S., & Inslegers, R. (2015). Research on Balint groups: A literature review. *Patient Education and Counseling*, *98*(6), 685–694. https://doi.org/10.1016/j.pec.2015.01.014

Vogel, L. (2018, October 29.). Even resilient doctors report high levels of burnout, finds CMA survey. *Canadian Medical Association Journal*, *190*(43), E1293. https://doi.org/10.1503/cmaj.109-5674

Walker, A. (2017, September 28). Suicide in nursing: Much more common than you think. Nurse.org. https://nurse.org/articles/suicide-rates-high-for-female-nurses/

Walton, A. (2018, April 3). Nordic countries continue to rank high in happiness, while America falls. *Forbes*. www.forbes.com/sites/alicegwalton/2018/04/03/nordic-countries-continue-to-rank-high-in-happiness-while-america-falls/#1957c76f23fa

Welp, A., Meier, L. L., & Manser, T. (2015). Emotional exhaustion and workload predict clinician-rated and objective patient safety. *Frontiers in Psychology*, *5*, 1573. https://doi.org/10.3389/fpsyg.2014.01573

Wible, P. (2018, October 10). 1103 doctor suicides & 13 reasons why. Pamela Wible MD: America's Leading Voice for Ideal Medical Care. www.idealmedicalcare.org/1103-doctor-suicides-13-reasons-why/

Wible, P. (2019, October 8). Why "happy" doctors die by suicide … (& how to prevent them). Pamela Wible, MD: America's Leading Voice for Ideal Medical Care. www.idealmedicalcare.org/preventing-happy-doctor-suicides/

Wignaraja, K., & Horvath, B. (2020). Universal basic income is the answer to the inequalities exposed by COVID-19. World Economic Forum. www.weforum.org/agenda/2020/04/covid-19-universal-basic-income-social-inequality/

World Bank (2018, September 19). Decline of global extreme poverty continues but slowed: World Bank. Press release. www.worldbank.org/en/news/press-release/2018/09/19/decline-of-global-extreme-poverty-continues-but-has-slowed-world-bank

World Health Organization (WHO) (2013). *Closing the health equity gap: Policy options and opportunities for action*. https://apps.who.int/iris/handle/10665/78335

World Health Organization (WHO) (2017, April 6–7). *Report of the policy dialogue meeting on the nursing workforce*. World Health Organization progress report. www.who.int/hrh/news/2017/NursingApril2017-2.pdf

World Health Organization (WHO) (2019). Year of the nurse and the midwife 2020. www.who.int/news-room/campaigns/year-of-the-nurse-and-the-midwife-2020

World Population Review (2020, April 6). Healthiest countries 2020. https://worldpopulationreview.com/countries/healthiest-countries/

Wu, B. (2018). The rise of Physician Assistant programs: How the physician shortage affects aspiring PAs. Barton Associates. www.bartonassociates.com/blog/the-rise-of-physician-assistant-programs-how-the-physician-shortage-affects-aspiring-pas

Wyatt, R., Laderman, M., Botwinick, L., Mate, K., & Whittington, J. (2016). Achieving health equity: A guide for health care organizations. IHI White Paper. Institute for Healthcare Improvement. Available at www.ihi.org

Zhang, Y., Han, W., Qin, W., Yin, H., Zhang, C., Kong, C., & Wang, Y. (2018). Extent of compassion satisfaction, compassion fatigue and burnout in nursing: A meta-analysis. *Journal of Nursing Management, 26*(7), 810–819. https://doi.org/10.1111/jonm.12589

Appendix A

THE TRANSFORMATIVE POWER OF LANGUAGE

Agents of oppression:

People who have had oppressor patterns/identity forcibly imposed on them from a very young age. Disconnection, isolation, and guilt are key forces that shape this identity, yet their inherent goodness and caring are indestructible.

Ally:

A person who stands visibly with oppressed groups in the fight against their oppression while also fighting for their own humanity. They are willing to make mistakes as they build friendships across racial and cultural lines, take action against oppression, acknowledge and address oppressor patterns within themselves and their group, and support the leadership of oppressed groups.

Anti-Blackness:

The deliberate and/or unconscious actions by individuals or institutions that target Black people for destruction. The brutality and inhumanity of anti-Blackness are being exposed, faced, and challenged on a global scale by people of all racial backgrounds unified in a movement to end anti-Blackness.

Anti-Racist:

A white person who is committed to becoming increasingly aware of the current and historical brutality of racism and has decided to follow the leadership of People of the Global Majority (Black, Indigenous, and People of Colour) in interrupting racism. Anti-racists seek to heal from the damaging effects of racism in their own lives by restoring their connections with People of the Global Majority and other anti-racists. They also seek connection with white people who are overtly racist by listening, loving, and lifting spirits so they too can heal from the damage of racism and reclaim their humanity as good, caring white people.

Assimilation:

Forced attempts to absorb and subordinate racial and cultural groups within a dominant population and to separate people from their racial and cultural identity and their sense of self and community. These attempts are challenged by the forces of integrity, indignation, and collaborative resistance that are inherent in racial and cultural pride.

Asylum seeker:

A displaced person who is fleeing their home country due to persecution, war, or the threat of violence and is seeking safety and international protection in another country with the unsinkable determination to receive their rightful status and protections as a refugee.

BIPOC:

A term to describe the alliance among Black, Indigenous, and People of Colour in undoing Native invisibility, anti-Blackness, systematic racism, and white supremacy.

Black Lives Matter:

A part of a global movement dedicated to dismantling white supremacy by building strong alliances to intervene against violence enacted upon Black communities. Black Lives Matter (BLM) unleashes Black creativity, innovation, and joy.

Careworn:

Dedicated but under-resourced health and social care practitioners who experience emotional, psychological, physical, and spiritual exhaustion from the demands of their work within the context of oppressive systems that value profit over people. Despite the many limitations in the systems in which they work, they care deeply for their clients and colleagues, save lives, and promote health and wellbeing to the best of their ability.

Climate justice:

The eradication of the disproportionate and grave consequences of climate change on communities of colour and poor people throughout the world and the achievement of sustainable, nurturing, generative, and life-affirming environments for all people and all living things.

Colourism:

A mechanism by white people to divide and conquer People of the Global Majority (Black, Indigenous, and People of Colour) by using the shade of their skin colour to pit them against each other. The closer one's skin colour is to white, the more one is valued, privileged, desired, accepted, and protected from anti-Blackness or being targeted for destruction. This tool attempts to foster contempt, derision, disgust, dehumanization within communities of colour to weaken any unity in the fight against white racism. Colourism is resisted by the love, respect, wisdom, and appreciation deeply rooted within the spirit and soul of People of the Global Majority.

Cross-cultural communication:

The process of appreciating similarities and differences in communication across racial and cultural groups and reaching for a mutual connection, understanding, and support.

Culture:

The ordinary and extraordinary behaviour, habits, language, and values or "way of life" of a particular group of people. This concept can be extended not only to ethnic groups, but also to identity groups related to gender, race, socioeconomic class, age, sexual orientation, religion, and disability. Occupational groups, such as doctors, nurses, factory workers, teachers, also tend to share norms and social behaviours that comprise a distinct culture or way of being.

Dismantling oppression:

To gradually and systematically take apart and obliterate the institutional forces that uphold the systematic mistreatment of groups of people while simultaneously re-creating and releasing liberatory forces in society.

Frontline workers and communities:

People most impacted by threats to health and the devastating consequences of climate change – Indigenous people, People of the Global Majority, poor/working-class people, and direct production workers. They are the first workers and communities that experience threats to their health and the devastation from climate change. Although they suffer its worst consequences, they are the critical human infrastructure and the key leaders in the fight for human and planetary health.

Genocide:

The deliberate and systematic destruction and eradication of Indigenous, ethnic, racial, and cultural groups, fuelled by greed and the insatiable desire to hoard and consume more resources by ruling elites. Propaganda and scapegoating are the mechanisms used by ruling elites to convince the working class that it is in their self-interest to engage in genocide towards a group different from them. When a group of people survives attempted genocide, ruling elites often attempt to enact genocide on their culture through forced assimilation, yet are met with unwavering resistance, unshakeable resilience, and indomitable pride.

Health and social care practitioners:

Frontline warriors who are educated and trained to address the damage and destruction to human health and wellbeing that results from accidents, birth defects, contagious and genetic diseases, environmental factors, and also from social inequities and institutionalized oppression. Despite the social and health care systems that exploit their caring, health and social care practitioners alleviate suffering and champion the health and wellbeing of people of all racial and cultural backgrounds.

Human transformation:

The creative process through which individuals, relationships, communities, organizations, and societies are re-shaped and lifted by the power of artful listening and the interplay of loving and flexible minds that build connections, promote healing, and support profound, everyday leadership towards creating a just and sustainable world.

Immigrant:

A person who is a permanent resident in a country other than that of their birth, because they hoped for a life with safety, financial security, access to basic needs, and meaningful community engagement and occupational participation.

Implicit bias:

Conscious and/or unconscious automatic thoughts that influence and lead to rigid and often hurtful responses towards other groups of people and their own group.

Increasing awareness of one's own implicit bias, coupled with healing relationships within and across racial and cultural lines, dispels preconceived ideas about racial and cultural identity groups and promotes flexible thinking and caring actions towards all people.

Intercultural communication:

The process of learning from, with, and about people from different racial and cultural groups that leads to a mutual and transformative experience.

Internalized oppression:

The internalization of invalidating messages, misinformation, and lies inflicted on oppressed groups about themselves, about their history, and about their stories that take root in the form of hate towards oneself and one's own group. Internalized oppression is contradicted and washed away in deeply caring listening partnerships within and across racial and cultural lines that support the release of tears, laughter, shaking, raging, and talking.

Intersectionality:

The convergence of multiple identities in oppressed people and groups that creates an interwoven and strong foundation for awareness, hope, human possibility, and deft action in the world.

Migrant:

A person who moves to a new location on a temporary basis. This may occur within the borders of one's own country or across borders. Forced migration due to devastating climate emergencies is increasing around the world and is disproportionately affecting People of the Global Majority. Migrants are often the engines of economies and share the magnificence of their cultures in their new locations.

Multicultural:

The existence of diverse racial and cultural groups within a group, organization, community, or population. Whenever multicultural groups resist assimilation and retain, celebrate, and share their cultures and languages, everyone they are in contact with and society as a whole are transformed.

Oppression:

The blatant and insidious one-way mistreatment and subordination of one group of people by another group of people acting as agents of oppression and/or by societal institutions. Each inflict unjust, cruel, harsh, and often deadly abuse of power, violence, and control over particularly targeted groups in society (see also "Dismantling oppression" above).

People of the Global Majority:

Also known as Black, Indigenous, and People of Colour. They are the racial majority in the world and will be the racial majority in the United States by 2050.

Pre-existing condition:

The historical and ongoing destructive forces within communities and populations who live with the chronic and ravaging experiences of oppressive systems which take an enormous toll on their minds, bodies, and spirits. These forces are rebuffed by the indomitable and invincible racial and cultural strengths inherent within these communities and populations and within their deep ties to each other and the Earth.

Prejudice:

Preconceived negative thoughts and feelings towards a person or group based on their racial or cultural identity (see "Implicit bias" above for transforming prejudice).

Racial and cultural fluidity:

The ability to respond flexibly and synergistically to diverse racial and cultural groups.

Racial and cultural humility:

A process allowing for recognition that there is much we don't know or understand about diverse racial and cultural groups and that mistakes are inevitable as we reach to connect across racial and cultural lines.

Racially and culturally effective communication:

The artful interplay between listening, speaking, and caring coupled with awareness, sensitivity, appreciation, and responsiveness to verbal and non-verbal communication and emotions while welcoming racial and cultural diversity and supporting connection, understanding, and mutually successful outcomes.

Racism:

The blatant and insidious one-way mistreatment and subordination of People of the Global Majority (Black, Indigenous, and People of Colour) by white people and/ or white-dominated societal institutions that inflicts unjust, cruel, harsh, and often deadly abuse of power, violence, and control over people based on skin colour and facial features. The unwavering progress humans have made towards ending racism in the past 60 years (since the civil rights movement in the United States in the 1960s) spell its eventual and inevitable doom and this will undeniably bring about a better world for all humans.

Refugee:

A person who has fled their country because of persecution, war, conflict, or the threat of violence and has been granted asylum and protection under international laws and conventions in another country. They have the opportunity to become lawful permanent residents in their new homeland and to contribute powerfully to the racial and cultural fabric of their new home.

Targets of destruction:

People who experience both blatant and insidious one-way mistreatment and subordination by people acting as agents of oppression and/or societal institutions that inflict unjust, cruel, harsh, and often deadly abuse of power, violence, and control over their identity group (see "Dismantling oppression" above).

Treasuring All Life:

A movement dedicated to engaging people of all ages and backgrounds in conversations about how to help the living Earth. People are supported in taking turns listening to each other and loving each other even if they disagree about environmental and racial justice. They are also taught the skills of lifting spirits as they identify steps to save our imperilled planet.

When you can:

Life presents limitless barriers and opportunities to engage in listening, loving, and lifting spirits within and across racial and cultural lines. Each time you, as a health or social care practitioner, are able to listen, love, and lift spirits with a client, colleague, co-worker, or within a health or social care team, synergistic contributions are made towards a hopeful transformation of the health and well-being of individuals, communities, and the planet.

White people:

People of European heritage who have been told they are white and have had racist patterns forcibly imposed on them from a very young age. Disconnection, isolation, and guilt are key forces shaping this identity, yet their inherent goodness and caring are indestructible.

White supremacy:

A system of norms, values, and beliefs that white people are superior to Black people, Indigenous people, and People of Colour. It is a system of belief that embodies the idea that the closer your skin colour is to white, the more you are valued and cherished, and the closer you are to Black, the more you are despised and reviled. White supremacy is enacted in hierarchical structures that are embedded in every institution within some societies. The flawed assumptions of genetic and cultural superiority, and rightful dominance, which reinforces separation primarily into white only and Black only societies, are being thoroughly challenged in this historic period of worldwide action within the BLM movement to eradicate racial injustice directed at Black people.

Appendix B

ASSESSING YOUR STRENGTHS AND AREAS FOR IMPROVEMENT AS A RACIALLY AND CULTURALLY EFFECTIVE COMMUNICATOR

Table B.1: Froehlich Communication Survey
Table B.2: Froehlich Communication Survey: Brief Version
Table B.3: Treasuring the Human Race Survey
Table B.4: Racial and Cultural Awareness and Action Survey
Table B.5: Treasuring All Life Survey

Table B.1 Froehlich Communication Survey

Name_____

Developing effective interpersonal communication is an ongoing process. The purpose of this survey is to help you identify your strengths, areas for improvement, and goals related to effective interpersonal communication. Please circle the number that best reflects your agreement with the following statements so you can clarify where you need to work to be a more effective communicator.

1	**Strongly Disagree**	**Much Improvement Needed**
	Disagree	**Moderate Improvement Needed**
	Agree	**Some Improvement Needed**
10	**Strongly Agree**	**Little Improvement Needed**

I can listen without interrupting.

1   2   3   4   5   6   7   8   9   10

I can keep my mind free of distractions while listening.

1   2   3   4   5   6   7   8   9   10

I can allow for silences.

1   2   3   4   5   6   7   8   9   10

When appropriate, I can offer steady eye contact while listening.

1   2   3   4   5   6   7   8   9   10

I am aware of body language while listening.

1   2   3   4   5   6   7   8   9   10

My posture and facial expression show interest and caring.

1   2   3   4   5   6   7   8   9   10

I don't fidget while listening.

1   2   3   4   5   6   7   8   9   10

I can build rapport with others.

1   2   3   4   5   6   7   8   9   10

I appropriately maintain confidentiality.

1   2   3   4   5   6   7   8   9   10

I can maintain compassion while listening.

1   2   3   4   5   6   7   8   9   10

I use open- and closed-ended questions to determine someone's concerns and goals.

1   2   3   4   5   6   7   8   9   10

I can effectively use restatement, summaries, and clarification in a conversation.

1   2   3   4   5   6   7   8   9   10

I can identify, reflect, and validate emotional and verbal content in a conversation.

1   2   3   4   5   6   7   8   9   10

I can maintain mental focus and support emotional release when listening to someone who is upset.

1   2   3   4   5   6   7   8   9   10

I can convey hopefulness.

1   2   3   4   5   6   7   8   9   10

I can use humor effectively.

1   2   3   4   5   6   7   8   9   10

I can judge when to use touch during conversations.

1   2   3   4   5   6   7   8   9   10

I can judge when to redirect someone or help someone get their attention off their distress in a conversation.

1   2   3   4   5   6   7   8   9   10

I can judge when someone is ready to hear information or advice.

1   2   3   4   5   6   7   8   9   10

I am clear, concise, and confident when I speak.

1   2   3   4   5   6   7   8   9   10

I can give, receive, and solicit constructive feedback including appreciation of others and myself.

1   2   3   4   5   6   7   8   9   10

I can be appropriately assertive in interactions with others.

1   2   3   4   5   6   7   8   9   10

I communicate well on teams by listening to multiple perspectives and sharing mine.

1   2   3   4   5   6   7   8   9   10

I understand the importance of seeking an interpreter when I don't understand the language of a client.

1   2   3   4   5   6   7   8   9   10

I can communicate effectively with people from different racial and cultural groups.

1   2   3   4   5   6   7   8   9   10

Score /250

Communication skills I want to be better at: (Progress reported on goals in post-survey)

1.

2.

3.

Additional Comments:

Thanks for your time.

Table B.2 Froehlich Communication Survey: Brief Version

Name_____

Developing effective interpersonal communication is an ongoing process. The purpose of this survey is to help you identify your strengths, areas for improvement, and goals related to effective interpersonal communication. Please circle the number that best reflects your agreement with the following statements so you can clarify where you need to work to be a more effective communicator.

1 Strongly Disagree   Much Improvement Needed
10 Strongly Agree   Little Improvement Needed

I can listen without interrupting.
1   2   3   4   5   6   7   8   9   10
I can keep my mind free of distractions while listening.
1   2   3   4   5   6   7   8   9   10
I can allow for silences in a conversation.
1   2   3   4   5   6   7   8   9   10
I am aware of body language while listening (i.e. eye contact, not fidgeting, facial expression).
1   2   3   4   5   6   7   8   9   10
I can build rapport and maintain compassion in conversations (i.e. greeting, tone of voice).
1   2   3   4   5   6   7   8   9   10
I can maintain mental focus when listening to someone who is upset.
1   2   3   4   5   6   7   8   9   10
I can effectively use clarification, validation, and summarizing in a conversation.
1   2   3   4   5   6   7   8   9   10
I am clear and concise when I speak.
1   2   3   4   5   6   7   8   9   10
I communicate well on teams by listening to multiple perspectives and sharing mine.
1   2   3   4   5   6   7   8   9   10
I communicate effectively with people different from me and seek an interpreter when necessary.
1   2   3   4   5   6   7   8   9   10

Score /100

Communication skills I want to be better at: (Progress reported on goals in post-survey)

1.
2.
3.

Additional Comments:

Thanks for your time.

Table B.3 Treasuring the Human Race Survey

Name_____

Treasuring the human race is a transformational, creative, and liberating process. The purpose of this survey is to help you notice your complete goodness as a human and identify goals related to racial/cultural awareness, competence, and humility. Please circle the number that best reflects your awareness and appreciation of different racial groups so you can identify action steps to take on your journey towards embracing racial diversity.

1 Strongly Disagree	Much Improvement Needed
10 Strongly Agree	Little Improvement Needed

I am aware of **my own ethnic heritage** (national origin of my ancestors).

1   2   3   4   5   6   7   8   9   10

I am aware of **why my ancestors came to this country o**r if I am Indigenous, I am aware of **my tribal heritage**.

1   2   3   4   5   6   7   8   9   10

I am aware of the historical context, strengths, and challenges of being an **immigrant** in my country.

1   2   3   4   5   6   7   8   9   10

I am aware of the historical context, strengths, and challenges of being a **refugee** in my country.

1   2   3   4   5   6   7   8   9   10

I am aware of **my own racial heritage**.

1   2   3   4   5   6   7   8   9   10

I am aware of the historical context, strengths, and challenges of being:

Indigenous or Native American Heritage

1   2   3   4   5   6   7   8   9   10

African Heritage

1   2   3   4   5   6   7   8   9   10

Asian Heritage

1   2   3   4   5   6   7   8   9   10

Arab Heritage

1   2   3   4   5   6   7   8   9   10

Latina/Latino/Latinx Heritage

1   2   3   4   5   6   7   8   9   10

Pacific Island Heritage

1   2   3   4   5   6   7   8   9   10

White European Heritage

1   2   3   4   5   6   7   8   9   10

I am aware of the historical context, strengths, and challenges of **speaking English as a second language**.

1   2   3   4   5   6   7   8   9   10

I attempt to **learn languages other than my first language**.

1   2   3   4   5   6   7   8   9   10

I am aware of **biases and prejudices within myself and my family** toward other racial groups.

1   2   3   4   5   6   7   8   9   10

I **refrain from acting on biases and prejudices** I have toward other racial groups.

1   2   3   4   5   6   7   8   9   10

I **value relationships with people from racial groups** different from my own.

1   2   3   4   5   6   7   8   9   10

I am comfortable **interacting with people from racial groups different from my own**.

1   2   3   4   5   6   7   8   9   10

I can **remember my goodness as a human even when I make mistakes** in interactions with people from different racial groups.

1   2   3   4   5   6   7   8   9   10

I **take action when I notice that someone is being hurtful or oppressive** to another human.

1   2   3   4   5   6   7   8   9   10

Score _____/200

What did you learn about yourself completing the survey?

Three steps I can take to further develop my ability to treasure the human race:

1.

2.

3.

Additional Comments:

Thanks for your time.

Table B.4 Racial and Cultural Awareness and Action Survey

Name_____

The journey toward racial and cultural competence is a deeply enriching process that is fueled by building relationships with people from diverse backgrounds. The purpose of this survey is to help you identify your strengths, areas for improvement, and goals related to racial and cultural awareness, racial and cultural humility and racial and cultural effectiveness. Please circle the number that best reflects your agreement with the following statements so you can clarify action steps you need to take to become increasingly racially and culturally aware and effective in building relationships across racial and cultural lines.

1 Strongly Disagree   Much Improvement Needed
10 Strongly Agree   Little Improvement Needed

I am **aware that culture encompasses many human experiences** related to race, gender, class, ethnicity, disability status, sexual orientation, religion, etc.

1   2   3   4   5   6   7   8   9   10

I am aware of **my own ethnic heritage** (national origin of my ancestors).

1   2   3   4   5   6   7   8   9   10

I am aware of **why my ancestors came to this country** or if I am Indigenous, I am aware of **my tribal heritage**.

1   2   3   4   5   6   7   8   9   10

I am aware of the historical context, strengths, and challenges of being an **immigrant** in my country.

1   2   3   4   5   6   7   8   9   10

I am aware of the historical context, strengths, and challenges of being a **refugee** in my country.

1   2   3   4   5   6   7   8   9   10

I am aware of the historical context, strengths, and challenges of being:

Indigenous or Native American Heritage

1   2   3   4   5   6   7   8   9   10

African Heritage

1   2   3   4   5   6   7   8   9   10

Asian Heritage

1   2   3   4   5   6   7   8   9   10

Arab Heritage

1   2   3   4   5   6   7   8   9   10

Latina/Latino/Latinx Heritage

1   2   3   4   5   6   7   8   9   10

Pacific Island Heritage

1   2   3   4   5   6   7   8   9   10

White European Heritage

1   2   3   4   5   6   7   8   9   10

Jewish or Jewish Heritage

1   2   3   4   5   6   7   8   9   10

Catholic or Catholic Heritage

1   2   3   4   5   6   7   8   9   10

Muslim or Muslim Heritage

1   2   3   4   5   6   7   8   9   10

Buddhist or Buddhist Heritage

1   2   3   4   5   6   7   8   9   10

Protestant or Protestant Heritage

1   2   3   4   5   6   7   8   9   10

Hindu or Hindu Heritage

1   2   3   4   5   6   7   8   9   10

Atheist or agnostic

1   2   3   4   5   6   7   8   9   10

Currently raised poor/working class

1   2   3   4   5   6   7   8   9   10

Currently or raised middle or professional class

1   2   3   4   5   6   7   8   9   10

Currently or raised upper class

1   2   3   4   5   6   7   8   9   10

Homeless person

1   2   3   4   5   6   7   8   9   10

Female

1   2   3   4   5   6   7   8   9   10

Male

1   2   3   4   5   6   7   8   9   10

Gay

1   2   3   4   5   6   7   8   9   10

Lesbian

1   2   3   4   5   6   7   8   9   10

Bisexual

1   2   3   4   5   6   7   8   9   10

Transgendered, Queer, Intersex, Non-Binary

1   2   3   4   5   6   7   8   9   10

A person with a visible disability

1   2   3   4   5   6   7   8   9   10

A person with a hidden disability

1   2   3   4   5   6   7   8   9   10

Large person

1   2   3   4   5   6   7   8   9   10

Stigmatized with mental illness

1   2   3   4   5   6   7   8   9   10

Older adult

1   2   3   4   5   6   7   8   9   10

Adult

1   2   3   4   5   6   7   8   9   10

Parent

1   2   3   4   5   6   7   8   9   10

Young adult (approximately 21–30)

1   2   3   4   5   6   7   8   9   10

Teen (approximately 13–20)

1   2   3   4   5   6   7   8   9   10

Young person (12 and under)

1   2   3   4   5   6   7   8   9   10

Speaking English as a second language

1   2   3   4   5   6   7   8   9   10

I attempt to **learn languages other than my first language**.

1   2   3   4   5   6   7   8   9   10

I am aware of **biases and prejudices within myself and my family** toward other groups.

1   2   3   4   5   6   7   8   9   10

I **refrain from acting on biases and prejudices** I have toward other groups.

1   2   3   4   5   6   7   8   9   10

I **value relationships with people from cultures** different from my own.

1   2   3   4   5   6   7   8   9   10

I am comfortable **interacting with people from groups different from my own**.

1   2   3   4   5   6   7   8   9   10

I can **remember my goodness as a human even when I make mistakes** in interactions with people from different racial and cultural groups.

1   2   3   4   5   6   7   8   9   10

I **take action when I notice that someone is being hurtful or oppressive** to another human.

1   2   3   4   5   6   7   8   9   10

I am **aware of the impact of sociocultural determinants and poverty on health**.

1   2   3   4   5   6   7   8   9   10

I **understand that listening to different viewpoints does not mean I agree**.

1   2   3   4   5   6   7   8   9   10

Score _____/500

Three action steps I can take to further develop my cultural knowledge, awareness, and effectiveness:

1.

2.

3.

Additional Comments:

Thanks for your time.

Table B.5 Treasuring All Life Survey

Name_____

Treasuring all life is the moral imperative of joining together within and across racial and cultural lines to honor, preserve, sustain, and restore all life on the planet. Treasuring all life is a transformational, creative and liberating process. The purpose of this survey is to help you notice your complete goodness, intelligence, and power as a human and to identify goals related to treasuring all life. Please circle the number that best reflects your awareness and appreciation of sustaining all life so you can join within and across racial and cultural lines to take action towards the flourishing of all life.

1 Strongly Disagree   Much Improvement Needed
10 Strongly Agree   Little Improvement Needed

I understand the importance of treasuring each and every form of life on planet earth.

1   2   3   4   5   6   7   8   9   10

I understand that cherishing every human within and across racial and cultural lines will assist us in the loving stewardship of all life on the planet.

1   2   3   4   5   6   7   8   9   10

I am aware that divisions between racial and cultural groups in society interfere with efforts to ensure the flourishing of all life.

1   2   3   4   5   6   7   8   9   10

I am aware of the importance of taking action to transform climate change.

1   2   3   4   5   6   7   8   9   10

I am aware of the disproportionate impact of climate change on racially and culturally diverse communities.

1   2   3   4   5   6   7   8   9   10

I am hopeful that humans can unite within and across racial and cultural lines to preserve and sustain all life.

1   2   3   4   5   6   7   8   9   10

I am aware of the significance of each and every species to the quality of my life and all life on earth.

1   2   3   4   5   6   7   8   9   10

I allow myself and support others to feel deeply as we face the mass extinction of precious species that is currently happening.

1   2   3   4   5   6   7   8   9   10

I am aware of the tremendous human innovations across racial and cultural lines that attempt to sustain all life.

1   2   3   4   5   6   7   8   9   10

I am proud of any and all action I and other humans take to preserve, restore, and sustain all life.

1   2   3   4   5   6   7   8   9   10

I refrain from blaming myself and others for climate change in favor of
joining others within and across racial and cultural lines and taking action
in the present.

1   2   3   4   5   6   7   8   9   10

I can remember the inherent goodness, intelligence, and power of all
humans as we join together within and across racial and cultural lines to
stop the increasing destruction of the planet.

1   2   3   4   5   6   7   8   9   10

I will back racial and cultural communities most affected by climate change.

1   2   3   4   5   6   7   8   9   10

I will combat the human tendency that longs for more and more material
resource.

1   2   3   4   5   6   7   8   9   10

I am aware that with rational and loving thought and action, there is enough
resource on earth to permit the flourishing of all life without damaging
the planet.

1   2   3   4   5   6   7   8   9   10

I will engage with others within and across racial and cultural lines to envision alternative economic systems that nurture, honor, and sustain the
wellbeing and interconnection of all humans and the planet.

1   2   3   4   5   6   7   8   9   10

I understand that having the material advantage over others, places people
in a position to contribute their advantage towards the restoration and
preservation of the living earth.

1   2   3   4   5   6   7   8   9   10

I commit to lovingly and powerfully intervening when others engage in
destructive actions toward humans and the living earth.

1   2   3   4   5   6   7   8   9   10

I will take immediate steps both large and small with others within and
across racial and cultural lines to prevent further destruction of the planet.

1   2   3   4   5   6   7   8   9   10

I am willing to feel and face uncomfortable emotions as I join with others
within and across racial and cultural lines to take action to sustain all life.

1   2   3   4   5   6   7   8   9   10

Score _____/200

What did you learn about yourself from completing the survey?

Three steps I can take to further treasure all life:

1.

2.

3.

Additional Comments:

Thanks for your time.

Appendix C

LISTENING AND ENGAGING TO TRANSFORM

Listening partnership questions and discussion/journal prompts

Table C.1 Partnerships on the art of effective communication within and across racial and cultural lines

Adapted from: Froehlich, J. (2017). "Effective communication". In K. Jacobs & N. MacRae (Eds), *Occupational therapy essentials for clinical competence* (3rd ed., pp. 106–107; 110). Thorofare, NJ: SLACK, Inc.

Listening partnerships

Listening partners take turns exchanging engaged listening with each other. In the first listening exchange of 1 minute each way, it is recommended that the listener say nothing. This will sensitize listening partners to the tendency to interrupt others, strengthen their ability to listen without interrupting, and increase awareness of the significance of non-verbal communication. In all other partnerships, the listener is

TABLE C.1.I Presence and attunement (Chapter 3)

Listening and beyond: Dimensions of engaged listening	Questions for dialogue and connection *Each speaker decides on which question(s) they would like to answer*	Journal/discussion prompts
Presence Mind free of distractions Not interrupting Allowing for silences (1 minute each way – listener says nothing) ★This is the only listening partnership where the listener says nothing.	Consider your racial and cultural background as you answer these questions: • What were communication patterns like in your family of origin? • Are you more comfortable listening or speaking? • What is it like to allow for silences? • Why do you want to be a health or social care practitioner?	1. What was it like to listen and be listened to for 1 minute without interrupting? 2. Discuss if you would have preferred more or less time and for your partner to say something? 3. What kind of non-verbal communication did you use? 4. What helps you keep your mind free of distractions when listening? 5. Was culture or race a factor in your experience of listening without interrupting?
Attunement Eye contact Body language Posture and facial expression Fidgeting (2 minutes each way)	• What have you noticed about the non-verbal communication of people from different racial and cultural backgrounds? • What have you noticed about your non-verbal communication? Can you sit still or do you fidget? • What is it like to make eye contact as a listener or a speaker? • Have there been times when you did not feel listened to because of someone's non-verbal behaviour? • Talk about how technology affects non-verbal communication.	6. Was this listening partnership any easier than the first one? 7. Were you conscious of your non-verbal behaviour, as you were the listener? 8. What did your partner do well in terms of non-verbal communication? 9. Would it be useful to practise different facial expressions in front of a mirror or use a video recording to develop more awareness of flexibility? 10. Discuss if you have been able to continue practising not interrupting.

TABLE C.1.II Loving and inviting life narratives (Chapter 4)

Listening and beyond: Dimensions of engaged listening	Questions for dialogue and connection Each speaker decides on which question(s) they would like to answer	Journal/discussion prompts
Love and caring Build rapport Confidentiality Compassion (3–5 minutes each way)	Describe experiences with love, caring, rapport building, and compassion with people from diverse racial and cultural backgrounds. • What does the word respect mean to you? Is it possible to respect people you do not like? • What do the words love and caring mean to you? Do caring and love have a place in health or social care? • What does compassion mean to you? Empathy? • Talk about confidentiality in listening partnerships and other relationships.	1. What went well in this listening partnership? 2. What could have made it even better for both individuals? 3. Discuss if there was an opportunity to allow for silence. 4. What helps build rapport and convey compassion within and across racial and cultural lines? 5. Discuss what it was like to share your life experiences from the lens of your racial and cultural background. 6. What was it like to share news and goods as well as challenges and/or concerns with a listening partner? 7. Reflect upon your use of open- and close-ended questions. 8. What did you learn about yourself by sharing and listening to life stories with each other? Discuss any racial and cultural differences that emerged. 9. Where was the most emotion in this exchange? Were you able to delve into the topic that brought up the most emotion? 10. What was it like to share goals with each other? 11. Discuss the relevance of asking questions to understand key concerns and goals in your future practice. 12. What made listening partnerships on your current concerns, goals and, life stories go well and what could have made them go even better?
Inviting life narratives Asking questions – news and goods/ concerns and challenges (10+ minutes each way) **Life stories and life goals** (15+ minutes each way)	Share your life experiences from the lens of your racial and cultural background: • What is new and good in your life? • What is hard or challenging in your life right now? Or where do you need a hand? Tell me more. • Discuss what would increase your comfort level in sharing your life story with people from different racial and cultural backgrounds. • What are some pleasant memories of being a child within your family, neighbourhood, school, church or community? • What was difficult or challenging in your childhood? • What are some pleasant memories of your adolescence? • What was your favourite activity? What made you laugh and who did you laugh with? Talk about your first job. • What was difficult or challenging about being an adolescent? • Talk about what is great, what was or is challenging about being a young adult and/or adult? • What are your goals, both short- and long-term for the health and wellbeing of yourself, your family, your friends, your community, and the living Earth?	

TABLE C.1.III Aligning and responding to emotions (Chapter 5)

Listening and beyond: Dimensions of engaged listening	Questions for dialogue and connection / Each speaker decides on which question(s) they would like to answer	Journal / discussion prompts
Validation **Restatement** **Clarification** **Summaries** **Reflection** **Mental focus** **Supporting emotional release** (15+ minutes each way)	What is it like to align or connect with people within and across racial and cultural lines no matter how they present or how they are feeling? • How can you tell when you are aligned or not aligned with someone? • Talk about times when you felt validated or invalidated by a listener. • Talk about times when you offered your validation to someone. • Share what it is like to use restatement, clarification, validation, and summaries in difficult conversations. • Describe emotional expression in your family. Were there any gender differences in the expression of emotion? • Discuss any cultural or racial differences you have noticed in the expression of emotion. • What do you currently do when you feel upset? Is there anyone you can turn to if you need to cry? • What do you anticipate it will be like to listen to future clients when they share painful emotions?	1. Reflect upon how to strengthen your alignment with your listening partner or partners. 2. Identify your strengths and areas for improvement in using validation, restatement, clarification, and summaries as a listener. 3. Summarize what your listening partner shares and give each other feedback. 4. With whom do you feel comfortable venting your emotions? What would it take to feel comfortable venting to a listening partner? 5. What have you noticed about how you think and feel when you have had a chance to laugh, cry, shake, or rage? Have you been able to listen to someone when they cried hard? 6. Discuss what it is like to maintain mental focus when someone is upset. Can you do this when someone is upset with you? 7. Discuss which emotions are the easiest for you to listen to. 8. Are you able to stay in roles as a listener and a speaker in your listening partnerships?

TABLE C.1.IV Lifting spirits (Chapter 6)

Listening and beyond: Dimensions of engaged listening	Questions for dialogue and connection Each speaker decides on which question(s) they would like to answer	Journal/discussion prompts
Hopefulness **Humour** **Touch** **Redirection** **Attention off distress** **Advice/information** (15+ minutes each way)	Share experiences from within and across racial and cultural lines. • What makes you hopeful when you are discouraged? • What kind of humour lifts your spirits? Can you help others laugh to lift their spirits? • Does culture or race play a role in humour in your life? • Talk about the role of touch in health and social care and your comfort level with touch across and within racial and cultural groups. • Share a time when you were redirected or wanted to redirect someone and were or were not successful. • Talk about times when you helped someone, or they helped you get your attention off your distress. • Talk about times when you were given advice or information and it was or was not effective or welcome.	1. Discuss what it is like to maintain hopefulness and use humour and touch when listening. 2. What have you learned about adapting touch in COVID-19? 3. In your future practice, what do you anticipate it will be like to redirect or help clients from diverse racial and cultural backgrounds to get their attention off their distress and to celebrate the present? 4. Explore situations where it may be hard to redirect a client.

TABLE C.1.V Teamwork and collaboration (Chapter 7)

Listening and beyond: Dimensions of engaged listening	Questions for dialogue and connection — Each speaker decides on which question(s) they would like to answer	Journal/discussion prompts
Communicating across racial and cultural differences	• Talk about building relationships, communicating, and being on teams with people from different racial and cultural groups. What has gone well and what has been challenging?	1. Discuss what you can do to ensure that team members across racial and cultural lines, including yourself, each get a turn to share their perspective.
Interpreters, racial and cultural brokers	• Share any experiences you have had communicating with people who do not speak your first language.	2. Discuss experiences using interpreters and cultural brokers and what you know about racial and cultural literacy.
Health literacy	• Talk about experiences with learning a new language.	3. Discuss the goals you might have regarding learning new languages.
Clear and concise	• Talk about your strengths and areas for improvement in delivering clear and concise information.	4. Discuss any goals you might have regarding assertive, clear, and concise communication.
Asserting oneself	• Discuss situations in which your communication style is passive, passive-aggressive, assertive, or aggressive, and why?	5. What would help you welcome constructive feedback?
Giving and receiving feedback	• Share positive and negative experiences with receiving feedback.	6. Discuss whether you have been videotaped interacting with others and whether or not you are ready to implement this to improve your communication skills.
Conflict resolution	• What strategies can you employ to solicit constructive feedback?	7. Who can you turn to for support when you encounter a communication challenge?
Roles and responsibilities	• Describe any communication challenges you have faced relating to aggression, power dilemmas, resistance, avoidance, etc. What did you do that was effective and what would you do differently in the future?	8. What has it been like to offer support to a peer around communication challenges?
Appreciation (15 + minutes each way)	• Discuss the influence of culture or race in communication challenges you have experienced.	9. Discuss a conflict you did not handle well and identify how you might handle it differently now.
	• What is challenging for you in situations of conflict? How would you like to handle conflict differently? Discuss the influence of culture and race, and if they are factors in how you handle conflict.	10. Discuss the potential role of taking turns at listening to resolve conflict.
	• How was conflict handled in your family as you were growing up?	11. What is it like to appreciate yourself and others?
	• Talk about times when you successfully handled conflict.	
	• Share appreciations of yourself and your listening partner.	

encouraged to mostly listen, but to go beyond listening and fully engage as they encourage partners to share their experiences within and across racial and cultural lines. The following potential questions and suggested time frames for the exchange of listening walk listening partners through the process of cultivating the many dimensions of racially and culturally effective communication: presence, attunement, love, and respect, inviting the sharing of life stories, aligning and responding and lifting spirits. Keeping a perspective on each other's common humanity, while at the same time acknowledging and appreciating the influence of racial and cultural identity, will enhance listening partnerships, discussions, and journalling.

Table C.2 Partnerships to support understanding racial and cultural identities and experiences with oppression

Adapted from: Froehlich, J. (2017). "Effective communication". In K. Jacobs & N. MacRae (Eds), *Occupational therapy essentials for clinical competence* (3rd ed., pp. 108–109). Thorofare, NJ: SLACK, Inc.

TABLE C.2.I Partnerships for understanding oppression and internalized oppression within and across racial and cultural lines (Chapter 8)

| Listening to understand racial and cultural identities and experiences with oppression | Questions for dialogue and connection
Each speaker decides on which question(s) they would like to answer | Journal/discussion prompts |
|---|---|---|
| **Oppression and internalized oppression across and within racial and cultural lines**

(15+ minutes each way) | • What is your cultural, racial and ethnic background?
• What are you proud of and what are challenges related to your racial, cultural heritage, and ethnic heritage?
• Were you ever a member of a cultural or racial minority in your neighbourhood, school, church, or social situation as you were growing up? If so, what was this like?
• Were there ever times that you felt mistreated as a member of a particular group? What was this like?
• Discuss what it has been like to stand against the mistreatment of other racial and cultural groups.
• If you live in a country different from that of your ethnic origin, why did you or your ancestors come to the country you are living in now? Discuss if oppression was a factor.
• What makes you proud to be a citizen of _____ country and how would you like your country to be different?
• Discuss the results of several implicit bias tests with people from your own racial and cultural groups – what did you learn, what surprised you, and what action can you take to reduce your own implicit biases? | 1. What conditions enable you to open up about difficult experiences?
2. Discuss if you felt comfortable talking with your listening partner about times when you felt mistreated.
3. Discuss times you made friends with someone from a different racial, ethnic or cultural, group.
4. Discuss times when you have made mistakes in interactions with people from different ethnic, racial, and cultural groups.
5. What holds you back from building relationships across ethnic, racial, and cultural differences? What would help you take risks in building relationships across ethnic, racial, and cultural differences?
6. What is it like to have a dialogue about culture, race, and ethnicity?
7. Discuss a time when someone from a racial or cultural group different from your own pointed out a microaggression or oppressive behaviour you directed at them. How did you feel, how did you respond and share if you were able to learn from this experience? If so, what factors enabled you to learn from this experience? |

TABLE C.2.II Partnerships for understanding the relationship between oppression, health, and wellbeing (Chapter 9)

Listening to understand racial and cultural identities and experiences with oppression	Questions for dialogue and connection *Each speaker decides on which question(s) they would like to answer*	Journal/discussion prompts
Oppression and health (15+ minutes each way)	• What have you noticed regarding the social determinants of health in your family, friends, acquaintances, or people you have worked with? • Which health consequences of oppression for particular identity groups do you find the most moving, disturbing, or surprising? • What is your perspective on the oppression of males and do you agree that the societies we live in are oppressive towards boys and men, or not? • What does the wealth–health gradient mean for you personally? • What have you noticed or learned about climate change and health? How do you feel about it and what action would you like to take? • What helps you with feelings of discouragement? • Talk about resilience in yourself and others.	1. Complete the ACES Survey https://acestoohigh.com/got-your-ace-score/ and discuss or write in your journal about the meaning of your score. 2. Identify a racial or cultural group of which you would like to gain more knowledge and further explore the health challenges and health triumphs experienced by this group. 3. What action steps can you take to fight the health consequences of oppression?

Table C.3 Partnerships to build alliances and pride within and across racial and cultural lines

TABLE C.3 Partnerships to build alliances and pride within and across racial and cultural lines (Chapter 10)

Engaged listening to build alliances and pride within and across racial and cultural lines (15 minutes minimum each way on a selected identity)	Questions for dialogue and connection across all divisions (Members within constituency groups as well as allies across constituency groups will benefit from exchanging listening to the following questions. Speakers choose which questions they would like to address)
Strengthening natural alliances across gender	• What is magnificent about being _____? What is the truth about how phenomenal you are?
Women and girls as warriors	• What are you proud of about being _____?
Men and boys as close brothers	• What has been hard/difficult about being _____?
Transcending boundaries – Transgender, Intersex, Queer people, and your particular gender identity	• How have you been mistreated as a _____?
Collaborating with people of diverse sexual orientation	• What barriers have you had (or do you have) to overcome to have a great life as a _____?
Lesbians at the centre	• Where has _____ oppression impacted your life?
Gay men – whole and complete	• How has internalized oppression impacted your life?
Full inclusion of Bisexual people	• What is important for me to know about your life story? (Encourage us to feel grief, terror, confusion, self-doubt, and rage in telling our life story. Be open, interested, and eager to hear our triumphs and our hurts.)
Heterosexuals as allies to LGBTQ+ people	• What are you really like when _____ people are not around? What is it like to not have _____ around?
Embracing religions	
Cherished and esteemed Muslims	• What can _____ people do for you that would have the most immediate impact on your life?
Vital and loved Jewish people	• How can _____ people be your most trustworthy ally?
Warm and welcoming Christians	
Your particular religious/spiritual group as a healing force	
Valued atheists and agnostics	
Shedding class divisions	
Proud and brilliant raised poor/working-class world changers	
Proud and visible middle-class agents of change	
Fully human owning-class people	

(continued)

TABLE C.3 (Cont.)

Engaged listening to build alliances and pride within and across racial and cultural lines (15 minutes minimum each way on a selected identity)	Questions for dialogue and connection across all divisions (Members within constituency groups as well as allies across constituency groups will benefit from exchanging listening to the following questions. Speakers choose which questions they would like to address)
Treasuring the human race	• What is the most important thing you need to say to ____ people right now?
Beautiful and courageous people of African heritage	• What do you think that ____ people do not understand about being a ____ person?
Beloved and resilient people of Native/Indigenous heritage	• What do you want others to know about ____?
Caring, unified, and compassionate people of Pacific Island and Pilipino heritage	• How have you been an ally to people from constituency groups other than your own?
Delightful and wise Arab people	
Dignified and loving Asian heritage people (East, West, South, Central)	
Enduring and powerful people of Latino/a or Latinx heritage	
Good white European heritage people	
Universal humans – Multi-racial heritage people	
Loving humans across their life span	
Parents as shapers of a loving world	
Powerful young people	
Young adults as a key force	
Bold older people	
Honouring all shapes and abilities	
Elegant and essential people with disabilities	
Large and luscious people of size	
Mental health system and emotional trauma survivors	
Valiant navigators of recovery	
Celebrating national origin and ethnicity	
Glorious people of every ethnicity/national origin	
Unwavering and strong migrants, asylum seekers, and refugees	

Journal/discussion prompts

1. What did you learn about yourself that you did not know before these listening partnerships?
2. What did you learn from your partner(s) that will assist you in becoming an even more powerful ally to your own people or people of _____ heritage?
3. What are you looking forward to in your partnerships with _____?

Table C.4 Partnerships for deeper and restorative connections and understanding

Adapted from: Froehlich, J. (2017). "Effective communication". In K. Jacobs & N. MacRae (Eds), *Occupational therapy essentials for clinical competence* (3rd ed., pp. 108–109). Thorofare, NJ: SLACK, Inc.

TABLE C.4 Partnerships for deeper and restorative connections and understanding (Chapter 10)

Engaged listening to transform racial and cultural lines	Potential listening partnership questions Each speaker decides on which questions they would like to answer (15 minutes minimum each way on selected questions)	Journal/discussion prompts
Gender	• Tell your life story as a male or female as someone who did not or does not fit within binary gender identities. • Talk about your experiences as someone of your gender. • Share your vision of a world without gender oppression.	1. What is it like to have a dialogue about gender? 2. What is it like to be close to people of your own gender identity and people of other gender identities? 3. What do you think about the reality that there is no limit to the many creative ways of expressing ourselves as gendered beings?
Sex and sexual orientation	• While you were growing up, what attitudes were communicated to you about sex and sexual orientation by family, clergy, teachers, and friends? Were you able to talk openly with anyone? • Share your experiences with people of diverse sexual orientations. • If you feel comfortable doing so, talk about your experiences as someone of your sexual orientation.	4. What is it like to be close to people of your own sexual orientation? 5. If you have a friend who is LGBTQ+, what would it be like to ask them what it has been like to be his or her identity?
Class background	• Discuss your own class background. What did your parents and grandparents do for work? Did your family have enough, less than enough or more than enough? Did your class background change? • What are your earliest memories of noticing that someone had less than enough or more than enough? • Discuss if you have interrupted classism.	6. Discuss your feelings about talking about class and the feelings you have about classism. 7. Discuss your vision of a world where everyone has their basic needs met. 8. What would it be like to give up your privilege?

Disability

- Talk about a disability you currently have or an accident, injury, or disability you had in the past. Describe both positive and challenging aspects of your situation.
- Share your experiences, both positive and challenging, with people with disabilities.

9. What disability would be the hardest for you to have or to work with and why?
10. If you are able-bodied, discuss what it is like or would like to reach out and build friendships with people with disabilities?

Race

- Talk about your early memories of noticing people with a skin colour different from your own.
- How has racism affected you?
- What has enabled you to face the brutality of racism?
- What have you done to interrupt racism?
- What is it like to follow the lead of People of the Global Majority?
- If you are white, what is it like to get close to other white people who are overtly racist?

11. What is it like to have a dialogue about racism?
12. Share your vision of a world without racism.
13. What are your committed action steps towards dismantling racism?
14. Discuss what action steps you think white people should take towards making reparations for the enslavement of African Heritage people.
15. Discuss any mistakes you have made in getting close to people of a different race. Discuss the support needed to learn from these mistakes.

Size

- What do you appreciate about your own body?
- What factors limit your ability to completely appreciate your body and the bodies of others?
- Share thoughts about how to interrupt oppression based on size.

16. Discuss whether large women and men feel comfortable talking with you about their oppression.
17. What would help you appreciate your own body more?

Age

- Have you ever been mistreated for being a particular age?
- Talk about the age group you have the hardest time relating to and share your experiences with that group.

18. What concerns you about growing older?
19. How would you like to be treated as an elder?

(continued)

TABLE C.4 (Cont.)

Engaged listening to transform racial and cultural lines	Potential listening partnership questions Each speaker decides on which questions they would like to answer (15 minutes minimum each way on selected questions)	Journal/discussion prompts
Mental health	• What is your earliest memory of someone being described as crazy? • People are often labelled crazy when they have big feelings about the trauma and mistreatment they have endured. Discuss what you have noticed about this situation. • If you have received mental health services, what has been helpful, and what has not been helpful?	20. People who use mental health services are often stigmatized, jailed, homeless, and shunned by society. Discuss your awareness and experiences of this group that is often marked for destruction by society. 21. What have you noticed about human resiliency and the potential to recover from heavy trauma?
Religion/spiritual beliefs and heritage	• Describe your religious/spiritual heritage and current practices. • What are the strengths? Is there anything you wish was different about your religious heritage? • What has it been like to develop relationships with people of other religious/spiritual backgrounds?	22. What do you want to know about other religions or spiritual practices?
National origin and ethnicity	• Describe your ethnicity(ies) and national origin(s). • If you are not residing in your country of origin, why did you or your people locate to where you live now? • What is uniquely important that is offered by people of your ethnicity(ies) or national origin(s)? • Discuss if you are living on stolen land. If you are living on native land, how have your people personally benefitted from the genocide of Native/Indigenous people?	23. Discuss the pros and cons of assimilation into a new culture or nation. 24. Discuss what it would be like or steps you might take to further explore your national origin(s) and ethnicity. 25. Discuss what action steps you think should be taken to make reparations to Native/Indigenous people for stealing their land and resources.

Table C.5 Partnerships to support listening in health and social care teams: Voices of frontline workers as leaders

TABLE C.5 Partnerships to support listening in health and social care teams: Voices of frontline workers as leaders (Chapter 11)

Listening to each other as health and social care practitioners	Questions for dialogue and connection Each speaker decides on which questions they would like to answer (15 minutes minimum each way on selected questions)	Journal/discussion prompts
Pride	• What are you proud of and appreciate about your profession?	1. What stood out for you among practitioner responses, peer responses, and your own responses to the interview questions?
Challenges	• What is hard, difficult, or challenging about being or becoming a practitioner in your chosen field?	
Collaboration with other practitioners	• Share about another health or social care profession you have appreciated collaborating with.	
Listening, loving, and lifting spirits – within and across racial and cultural lines	• What have you noticed about listening, loving, and lifting spirits as a student health or social care practitioner? • What have you noticed about listening, loving, and lifting spirits within and across racial and cultural lines?	2. Discuss what it will be like to invite other health and social care practitioners to answer the interview questions.
Racial and cultural identity as a prac-titioner	• Discuss your perspective on the role of having others (peers, therapists, colleagues, partners) listen, love, and lift your spirits in your role as a _____.	3. What action steps would you like to take to enhance the health and wellbeing of all people and all living things?
Leadership	• Share how your racial and cultural identity has influenced you as a future practitioner.	
Giving and receiving feedback	• Discuss your experiences with collaboration and leadership. • What has supported the process of giving and receiving feedback to support the best practice as a student practitioner?	
Concerns	• What concerns you most as a future health or social care practitioner?	
Relationship between human and planetary health	• What do you see as the relationship between planetary health and human health?	
Hopes and visions	• What are your hopes and visions for a health care system that supports the flourishing of all racial and cultural groups – clients and practitioners alike? What has inspired this vision?	

Table C.6 Partnerships to embolden leadership

TABLE C.6 Partnerships to embolden leadership (Chapter 12)

Engaged listening to embolden leadership	*Questions for dialogue and connection* Each speaker decides on which question(s) they would like to answer (15 minutes minimum each way on selected questions)	*Journal/discussion prompts*
Leaders in your life **Your leadership**	• Discuss the traits you have admired in both inherent and designated leaders.	1. Identify goals for yourself as both an inherent and designated leader.
	• What specifically have you learned from leaders of different racial and cultural backgrounds that has affected your leadership?	2. What feelings do you need to overcome to take bold action?
	• Discuss examples of leadership within your family.	3. Share your experiences in making mistakes as a leader, what you learned, and how you have grown.
	• Discuss your experiences as an inherent leader and as a designated leader, and whether you had to overcome feelings of fear, inadequacy, or reluctance to lead.	4. Discuss times when you have effectively decided to follow rather than to lead.
	• Discuss your leadership or backing of leaders of diverse groups.	
	• What strengths do you bring to leadership roles and what challenges have you experienced?	
	• What are you most proud of as a leader?	
	• Discuss the support you have experienced or the lack thereof as a leader.	
	• Discuss your awareness of when it makes sense to lead and when it makes sense to follow.	

Appendix D

HEALTH AND WELLBEING OF PEOPLE UNDER THREAT

The health consequences of oppression are heartbreaking and unacceptable. Racism, sexism, homophobia, anti-Semitism, classism, other forms of oppression, and their multiple intersections inflict trauma, destroy lives, and limit the health and wellbeing of many groups of people. Yet, humans are resilient. The reader is invited to explore the damaging effects of systematic and institutional mistreatment of diverse groups of people while remembering that there are innumerable stories of people overcoming and triumphing over the consequences of oppression on their health and fulfilment in daily life. Below, alphabetically, are examples of the health consequences of oppression for many but not all oppressed groups. The reader is invited to continually seek more information on both the threats to human health and the extraordinary health victories of racial and cultural groups across the globe.

Africans, the original people: Our beautiful and courageous ancestors

Africans represent 70% of the world's poorest people. Many live on less than $1.90 per day (Hamel et al., 2019). With poverty comes poor health. The sub-Saharan African nations of Chad, the Central African Republic, Guinea, Liberia, and Benin are ranked as the countries with the lowest prosperity, poorest health, and poorest health care infrastructure in the world (Legatum Institute, 2018). Prior to the coronavirus pandemic, people in Africa were escaping poverty faster than people were moving into poverty (Hamel et al., 2019). Yet, without swift and effective action taken to increase health and economic resources in many poor regions in Africa, thousands of lives may be lost, and millions more people in sub-Saharan African may be pushed into extreme poverty in the pandemic (Mahler et al., 2020).

The United States is one of the most prosperous nations in the world, yet the legacy of racism in the United States yields stark health disparities across racial lines (Hammonds & Reverby, 2019). As we saw in Chapter 9, the risk of being killed by police violence is a leading cause of death among young Black men and women (Edwards et al., 2019). Over the course of their life, Black men are 2.5 times more likely to be killed by police than white men. For those that survive police violence, many health threats remain. The COVID-19 infection rate in the United States is more than three times higher in predominantly Black counties compared to predominantly white counties, and the death rate for predominantly Black counties is six times higher than in predominantly white counties (Yancy, 2020). The perfect storm of hypertension, diabetes, obesity, and cardiovascular disease places Black people at great risk for COVID-19. The damaging and inhumane conditions (racial stereotyping and profiling, poverty, housing density, high crime rates, and poor access to health care and healthy foods) under which Black Americans grow up, live, learn, work, and play are the social determinants of these COVID-19 risk factors (Yancy, 2020).

The leading cause of death worldwide is heart disease (Centers for Disease Control, 2019). However, in the United States, African Americans are 20% more likely to die from heart disease than non-Hispanic whites (U.S. Department of Health and Human Services Office of Minority Health, 2020) – tangible evidence of the heart-wrenching toll the heart knows and shows. African American men have the highest overall cancer incidence across five population groups and were more than two times more likely to die from stomach or prostate cancer than white men (American Cancer Society, 2019). While diabetics undergo 130,000 amputations each year in the United States, Black patients lose limbs at triple the rate of others (Goodney et al., 2013). Furthermore, African American parents live with the disheartening pain that odds are stacked against their children even before birth. The infant mortality rate for these families is more than twice that of non-Hispanic white ones. African American women's maternal mortality rate is more than ten times that of women in most other industrialized nations (Black Women's Roundtable, 2015).

Asians: Dignified and loving people of East, West, South, and Central Asia

The majority of the world's people, almost 60%, live within the vast continent of Asia. While prosperity and longevity is noted among the Asian nations of Japan, Singapore, and South Korea, 40% of the 766 million people living on less than $1.90 per day survive in Asian countries (Mihtra, 2018). Afghanistan, Yemen, and Nepal are the poorest of the Asian nations (Bada, 2018). The World Bank estimates that rapid population growth within the context of scarce resources has resulted in hunger and acute malnutrition for almost 70% of Asian women and children. Corrupt governments, natural disasters, war, and a history of colonization also contribute to the scarcity of resources and ultimately poor health across many Asian nations (Mihtra, 2018; Williams, 2016). Unless effective action is taken, COVID-19 is expected to push 16 million more Asians, 12 million of whom are Indian, into extreme poverty in 2020 (Mahler et al., 2020).

According to Dr Grace Ma, founding director of the Center for Asian Health in the United States, more than 70% of Asian Americans are foreign-born and many have limited English proficiency (National Institute on Minority Health and Health Disparities, 2016). Differing cultural beliefs and behaviours, unfamiliarity with the Western health system, and difficulty understanding instructions in a medical office are significant barriers to health care. Asian Americans experience health disparities in heart disease, hypertension, diabetes, and mental health, and unlike all other racial and ethnic groups in the United States, cancer is the leading cause of death in Asian Americans. They have the highest rates of the most preventable cancers (liver and stomach cancer) and the lowest cancer screening rates compared to other racial and ethnic groups which lead to being diagnosed with cancer at a later stage. Half of Asian Americans with diabetes are unaware they have the disease, and thus are more likely to develop type 2 diabetes compared to whites, despite having lower weight and body mass. Genetic and metabolic factors, diet, physical inactivity, and acculturation all contribute to diabetes in Asian Americans. Noting that suicide is a leading cause of death among Asian Americans, Ma dispels the myth that mental health challenges are rare in this population. Cultural norms against expressing emotional distress often result in emotional pain manifesting as symptoms in the body (National Institute on Minority Health and Health Disparities, 2016).

Asian Americans experience new threats to their mental and physical health and wellbeing in the pandemic as anti-Asian hate crimes have risen exponentially (Loffman, 2020). The website Stop AAPI Hate, created in response to the rise in anti-Asian sentiments in the United States, tracks incidents. Two-thirds of occurrences reported involve verbal harassment, nearly 10% were physical assaults, and some were directed at frontline health care workers risking their lives to battle the virus (Loffman, 2020). Despite the backlash towards Asian heritage people in the United States, it is notable that South Korea has been a global leader in mitigating the coronavirus pandemic (Ahn, 2020). In partnership with the health care system, the government provides protective equipment for all health care workers, extensive testing and isolating of infected individuals, and contact tracing. Additionally, the government covers all medical costs associated with COVID-19 for citizens and foreigners living in the country and has successfully fostered a culture of social distancing and wearing masks. Thoughtful and transparent actions by the government on behalf of the South Korean people have engendered trust and successful adherence to governmental health policies (Ahn, 2020).

Females: Women and girls as warriors

According to UN Women (2020), women and girls are disproportionately affected by poverty. Although they spend triple the time and energy of boys and men in looking after children and the household, they receive little to no compensation for their work. In fact, their labour costs them opportunities for education and earning power in the job market (UN Women, 2020). Additionally, patriarchal practices far too often cost girls and women their health and wellbeing. Poor females suffer from having less food and poorer sanitation than males, and females across the globe struggle to maintain their physical, mental, and emotional wellbeing in the face of gendered violence and sexual exploitation (Health Poverty Action, 2018; UN Women, 2020). Unfortunately, as the pandemic deepens economic and social stress, hardships experienced by women and girls are amplified (United Nations, 2020). Gender-based violence is increasing exponentially, unpaid care work has increased as women are called to care both for children out of school and older persons, and access to sexual and reproductive health services are declining.

Even in wealthier nations, sexism affects women's health in subtle and not so subtle ways. Lewis et al. (2019) analysed data on over 2 million patients in the United States who activated emergency services for chest pain or out-of-hospital cardiac arrest. They found that women received a lower percentage of recommended treatments than men. Men were more likely than women to receive aspirin for chest pain and were significantly more likely to be resuscitated in the event of cardiac arrest. The greatest difference was that women were significantly less likely to be taken to the hospital in ambulances using lights and sirens.

African American women are often challenged by the intersection of multiple oppressions including sexual objectification, racism, and gendered racism (the intersection of racism and oppressive sexual experiences). Carr et al. (2014) collected data on 144 African American women of lower socioeconomic status who sought some form of mental health treatment. Analysis of confidential surveys revealed that all three forms of oppression were related to more depressive symptoms, yet exposure to racist events uniquely predicted depressive symptoms in African American women.

Immigrants: Unwavering and strong migrants, asylum seekers, and refugees

Globally, one in seven people are migrants – 258 million are international migrants and 763 million are internal migrants (WHO, 2019a). Although the majority of migrants choose to leave their homeland for a better life, many migrants flee their homes because of famine, drought, unrest, or economic collapse (Rescue.org, 2018). Only those who are forcibly displaced due to armed conflict or persecution are eligible to seek asylum and refugee status in host nations (WHO, 2019a).

Lucas Guttentag, immigration law expert and senior immigration advisor at the Department of Homeland Security during the Obama administration, clarifies that more than 50% of migrants arriving at the southern border of the United States are fleeing almost unprecedented, horrific violence in the Northern Triangle countries of El Salvador, Guatemala, and Honduras (Guttentag & Driscoll, 2019). In the past, most migrants at the US southern border were Mexican men seeking opportunities in the United States. Unaccompanied minors and families from the Northern Triangle countries began to arrive in greater numbers in 2012 and are now 60% of the total, compared with 10% in 2012. This new reality is not addressed by the US border enforcement which treats Northern Triangle migrants as threats who should be jailed and deterred rather than as refugees seeking asylum. More than 75% of migrants from the Northern Triangle demonstrate a "credible fear" of persecution and therefore have a "significant possibility" of being eligible for asylum, yet many are not heard or fairly adjudicated due to an under-resourced asylum system (Guttentag & Driscoll, 2019).

Migrants and refugees across the world often face life-threatening conditions as they travel from their homelands – assaults, robbery, rape, murder, kidnapping, and torture for ransom, threats from traffickers, abduction by gangs, and drowning as they attempt to cross bodies of water (Shetty, 2019; UNHCR, 2018). Those who survive the harrowing journey often arrive in adjacent nations only to face distressing conditions in migrant facilities as they await immigration proceedings. Although there is significant variation in detention centres across nations, many are prison-like facilities (Skodo, 2017). They are notoriously overcrowded, lack nutritious food and sanitation, and often deny access to connections with family and with the outside world (Chotner, 2019; Skodo, 2017; Young, 2019). Furthermore, because social distancing is not possible in crowded facilities, COVID-19 is rampant among refugees (Corley, 2020).

Migrant workers, many of whom do the essential work of harvesting our crops, labouring in construction or manufacturing, and cleaning our homes and workspaces, also tend to live in crowded dormitories and thus are extremely vulnerable to the coronavirus (Connell, 2020).

Additionally, hostile policies in some host nations result in no legal protections or safety nets for the many migrants who have lost their jobs in the pandemic (Connell, 2020). Some migrant families choose not to seek health and social care, including food assistance, because they fear discrimination and punitive interactions with providers and officials at public agencies (Bernstein et al., 2019). Elevated levels of stress and trauma associated with dehumanizing detention conditions, fear of deportation, actual deportation, and separation from loved ones have profound and enduring negative consequences on the physical, mental, and emotional health of all migrants, particularly children and families (Chotner, 2019).

Indigenous inhabitants: Beloved and resilient people of Native heritage

Indigenous, Native, or Aboriginal populations have valiantly fought the forces of genocide and colonization for centuries. The struggle to retain their land, their languages, their cultures, and their existence is ongoing. They are about 370 million in number and reside in more than 90 countries. Indigenous people are about 5% of the world's population, but are 15% of the world's extreme poor

(Hall & Gandolfo, 2016). The devastating consequences of their oppression include lower life expectancy, high infant and child mortality, high maternal morbidity and mortality, heavy infectious disease loads, malnutrition, stunted growth, increasing levels of cardiovascular and other chronic diseases, substance abuse, and depression (Valeggia & Snodgrass, 2015). In the United States, American Indian/Alaska Natives (AI/AN) have the highest rates of suicide of any US racial or ethnic group and the rate has been on the rise since 2003 (Leavitt et al., 2018). Genocide, inflicted on Indigenous people from colonizers, has been internalized and become self-perpetuating (Poupart, 2003).

Long-standing health disparities resulting from colonization now place Native Americans at great risk of mortality from the coronavirus. The Navajo Nation includes areas of Arizona, Utah, and New Mexico. Health authorities for the Navajo Nation reported 4,071 positive cases and 142 deaths (Touchin, 2020). If it were a state, the Navajo Nation would rank first in the country for confirmed cases per 100,000 people – ahead of New York and New Jersey (Sternlicht, 2020). However, Navajo officials acknowledge that these numbers may be skewed by the high rates of testing (Touchin, 2020).

Extreme loss, trauma, and grief from pandemics are not new to Native Americans. Lacking immunity to European diseases, the measles and smallpox epidemics killed 70% or more of the Native population in the Americas when Europeans first settled upon their land, and a disproportionate number of Native people died in the 1918–1919 influenza pandemic (Ostler, 2020). For hundreds of years, Indigenous people have spoken out against the devastating consequences of human greed and ill-treatment of the environment, and even predicted the pandemic we now face (Nuwer, 2020). Some tribal leaders believe that the pandemic was unleashed by the unbalancing of the habitats of species through deforestation and commercial wildlife trade. Nuwer (2020) suggests that the pandemic is an opportunity to finally listen to Indigenous voices, follow their leadership, and adopt Indigenous-inspired ways of coexisting with nature.

Islamic people: Cherished and esteemed Muslims

Islam is the fastest-growing religion in the world and the number of Muslims in Europe and the United States is growing rapidly. According to the Global Terrorism Database, Muslims are the most likely victims of terrorist attacks. Although most of these attacks are in Muslim-majority nations, there appears to be an increase in attacks targeting Muslims in Europe and the United States (Herrera, 2019). There are currently about 3.45 million Muslims in the United States (Lipka, 2017). A poll by Mogahed and Chouhoud (2017) found that 60% of Muslims in the United States, more than any other religious group, reported religious discrimination. Muslim women reported more fear for their safety than Muslim men and indicated more emotional trauma. Although wearing the hijab can increase targeting for Muslim women, they are no more likely than men to change their appearance to be less identified as Muslim. Due to fear of community reaction and wanting to protect their partners and children, Muslim immigrant women are reluctant to call the police for domestic violence (Ammar et al., 2013). Muslims face both discrimination and lack of awareness of important religious considerations in health care – particularly conditions needed for prayer, the roles of medical treatment and religious authority, the importance of modesty, the religious concordance (shared identity) of clinicians, the role of the family in medical decision-making, advance care planning, and pain and symptom management (Boucher, 2017).

Nasim (2020) notes that the pandemic poses many hardships for Muslim people. Similar to the ultra-Orthodox Jewish community, social distancing is particularly hard because of the close-knit nature of many large Muslim families and the high frequency of religious gatherings. Even before the pandemic, Muslims in the UK were twice as likely to be in poverty than other people in Britain, and the virus is only worsening this economic disparity. Perhaps because the sanctity of human life is central in Islam, there is a disproportionate number of British Muslims in the medical field, and many have lost their lives in the line of duty. Nasim is hopeful that many Muslims are finding inspiration from the core Islamic values of patience, the sacrifice of wealth, and resistance to temptation as they navigate the loss of both lives and livelihoods and find generosity in these trying times.

Jews: Vital and loved children of Israel

The diaspora, or dispersal of Jews or Israelites out of their ancestral homeland, has led to the settlement of Jews across the globe. There are 16.6 million Jews worldwide (0.2% of the population), living mostly in Israel, the United States, Canada, France, and the UK. Ongoing acts of anti-Semitism, persecution, and scapegoating take a toll on the mental health and wellbeing of Jews. Loewenthal (2012) explored mental health and mental health care for Jews in the diaspora, with particular reference to the UK. Using demographic and psychiatric epidemiology, she found that the prevalence of depression may be as high among Jewish men as among women, yet the prevalence of anxiety, alcohol abuse, and suicide may be low by world standards. Jewish law generally forbids suicide, and this may explain lower suicide rates among Jews. Citing several studies, Loewenthal speculates that Jewish men may be labelled with depression more than non-Jewish men because they tend to be more willing to talk about their symptoms of depression and tend to refrain from moderate alcohol use, which may be used as an escape from depression in non-Jewish men. Additionally, because Jewish men are less violent, the incidence of domestic violence may be lower in Jewish homes, causing Jewish women to be less depressed and therefore equalizing rates of depression between Jewish men and Jewish women.

Ultra-orthodox Jews, or the Haredi community, in Israel, the United States, and the UK, have received media attention for resisting social distancing in the pandemic. On the surface, it appears that Haredi people are defying public health restrictions, yet Kasstan (2020) argues that long-running and unresolved relationships between Haredi communities and state officials are at the root of tensions in the pandemic. Differing views regarding health care are prominent in the discord. Haredim are stereotyped by state officials as "hard to reach" or "non-compliant" for historically refusing vaccines, and now for resisting social isolation measures. In reality, larger family sizes and strong familial and communal ties result in overcrowding and economic deprivation in the Haredi community. These factors contribute to the disproportionate COVID-19 related morbidity, hospital admissions, and deaths for Haredi people in Israel and the UK. Kasstan suggests that effective collaboration and strong communication between Haredi religious leaders and public health leaders must be achieved to break the stereotypes and protect the health of this growing minority community.

Large people: Large and luscious humans of size

Evidence shows that obese people experience discrimination, also known as sizeism, in employment settings, health care settings, educational settings, and within interpersonal relationships (Puhl & Heuer, 2009). Hutson (2017) proposes that because the human body, as seen in contemporary society, is viewed as both malleable (under our control) and intractable (an indicator of moral character), size discrimination remains basically unchallenged. For example, Puhl et al. (2008) found that individuals with a body mass index (BMI) of 30 or higher experienced employment discrimination at a rate of 5% for men and 10% for women – similar in effect to age and race discrimination. Additionally, assumptions between health and thinness have been found to be problematic. While findings from the Framingham Heart Study over a 24-year weight history show an association with maximum body mass index and mortality (Xu et al., 2018), Tian et al. (2020) found that all cause mortality in metabolically healthy individuals was not predicted by overweight and obesity.

Particularly harmful is "fat shaming" by well-intended health and social care practitioners. According to the American Psychological Association (2017), negative attitudes, microaggressions, and implicit bias towards large people among practitioners can cause stress and inhibit some clients from seeking medical treatment. Practitioner assumptions that weight is under an individual's control rather than the result of a confluence of societal factors, and the assumption that being fat means one is automatically unhealthy, pose a risk to the mental well-being of people who are overweight. Although many large and overweight people experience good health, both younger and older large and overweight people are at greater risk of contracting COVID-19 and thus deserve extra thought and care to reduce the prevalence of the coronavirus in this population (Kass et al., 2020).

Latin Americans: Enduring and powerful people of the Caribbean, South America, and Central America

Important declines in infant mortality, fertility rates, and prevalence of infectious diseases in Latin America and the Caribbean have occurred in the last decades

(Chelala, 2019). Latin America is now leading the world in decreasing infant mortality. Maternal mortality rates remain high as does the prevalence of HIV/ AIDS, malaria, dengue, tobacco and substance abuse, chronic non-communicable diseases, and mental disabilities. Many health problems on the rise are related to rapid urbanization, environmental problems, and rising income inequality. Levels of obesity are increasing across all ages, but particularly among children. Violence against women, including homicide by partners, has reached epidemic proportions in many Latin American countries and calls for new approaches to save lives and prioritize health and wellbeing for all (Chelala, 2019).

Public health infrastructure and preparedness for handling the coronavirus pandemic vary greatly across the nations of Latin America (Burki, 2020). While Ecuador has already seen a high death toll, Cuba has a health care system that is prepared and ready to respond. Venezuela's health care system has collapsed amid their humanitarian crisis, placing many lives at risk. Overcrowded prisons and slums across South and Central America prevent the social distancing required to limit the spread of the virus. Government officials have downplayed the seriousness of the virus in Brazil and Mexico, which will cost many lives (Burki, 2020).

In the United States, Hispanics and Latinos are the largest ethnic minority group. They have been the main drivers of US population growth since 2000. Hispanics of Mexican origin are the largest group followed by Puerto Ricans within the Hispanic population in the United States (Flores, 2017). Cancer is the leading cause of mortality among Hispanics, followed by cardiovascular diseases and unintentional injuries. Although the implementation of the Affordable Care Act of 2010 has resulted in improved access to health services for Hispanics, limited cultural sensitivity, health illiteracy, and a shortage of Hispanic health care providers are barriers to quality care, and many Hispanics remain uninsured. Despite lower socioeconomic status (SES) when compared with non-Hispanic whites, Hispanics tend to live longer than non-Hispanic whites, but this discrepancy may soon be offset by increasing rates of obesity and diabetes (Valasco-Mondragon et al., 2016).

Just as they are disproportionately frontline workers (grocery store staff, restaurant workers, caretakers, cleaners, and delivery workers), Latinos across the United States are disproportionately affected by the coronavirus – up to three times the rate of white Americans in some regions (Singh & Jirabm, 2020). Many have lost their frontline jobs in the pandemic, and only 38% of Latinos working in low-wage jobs have access to health coverage. Furthermore, US government policies and negative messaging about Latinos, leave many Latino immigrants feeling unsafe to seek care (Singh & Jirabm, 2020).

LGBTQ+: Breaking the limitations of gender identity and sexual orientation

According to the Global Forum (2017), consensual same-sex behaviour is criminalized in 72 countries. In 57 countries, transgender people are criminalized and prosecuted. Criminalization essentially blocks the right to health for many Lesbian, Gay, Bisexual, Transgender, Queer, and Intersex (LGBTQ+) people. Even in countries where same-sex marriage has been legalized, health disparities in LGBTQ+ individuals are prevalent. Key health concerns for the LGBTQ+ population include high rates of tobacco, alcohol and other drug use, homelessness among LGBTQ+ youth, mental health problems related to discrimination, high rates of sexually transmitted diseases among gay and bisexual men, health complications related to gender reassignment in transgender individuals, and decreased utilization of health care, particularly in rural areas where providers may have less knowledge, awareness, and skill in addressing LGBTQ+ health concerns (Shaver et al., 2018). Compounding the heavy oppression already experienced by LGBTQ+ people, targeting is worsening in the pandemic – particularly by law enforcement officials (Lavers, 2020).

According to the Office of the Surgeon General and National Action Alliance for Suicide Prevention (2012), compared to straight youth, lesbian, gay, and bisexual youth are five times more likely to attempt suicide. Equally disturbing, in a recent survey on adolescent attitudes and behaviours, more than half of transgender male teens, 29.9% of transgender females, and 41.8% of non-binary respondents stated they had attempted suicide at some point in their lives (Toomey et al., 2018). These rates of attempted suicide stand in stark contrast to rates for female adolescents (17.6%), and male adolescents (9.8%), and warrant strong interventions to build resilience among LGBTQ+ youth in the fight against family rejection, bullying, and harassment (Toomey et al., 2018).

Male humans: Men and boys as close brothers

The health disparities in the life span between those born female and those born male are noted worldwide. Prior to the coronavirus pandemic, females lived longer than males by up to 10 years in some countries (Regan & Partridge, 2013). High-risk behaviour, not seeking medical attention, exposure to occupational hazards, excessive drinking, and smoking are some of the factors that contribute to shorter life spans in males (Desjardins, 2004). Men's greater vulnerability to COVID-19 remains a mystery to the medical community, but there is speculation that lifestyle factors may contribute to the significantly higher rate of death seen in men compared to women in the pandemic (Walter & McGregor, 2020).

One could argue because men wield power in society and play an oppressive role towards women, that they themselves are not oppressed. Yet, how do we explain the robust health data existing even prior to the pandemic which showed that being male is not correlated with positive health outcomes (Baker et al., 2014)? Might men also be oppressed? New (2001) argues that men's human needs are not met within the gendered roles of modern society and men are systematically oppressed by the social construct of masculinity. Sex roles limit closeness, deny opportunities to share feelings, force engagement in high-risk behaviour, physical conflict, and war, and ultimately yield poor health and a shorter life span for men. Research shows that compared to girls, boys in the United States are more likely to be diagnosed with a behaviour disorder, prescribed stimulant medications, fail out of school, binge drink, commit a violent crime, and/or take their own lives (Representation Project, 2019).

Mental health system and emotional trauma survivors: Valiant navigators of recovery

Oppression is maddening. Yet the anger and righteous indignation felt by oppressed people is often pathologized and labelled. In fact, the mental health system has an ever-increasing set of diagnostic labels and psychiatric medications for the many ways humans exhibit thoughts, feelings, and behaviours. When humans show their distress in response to their trauma inflicted by poverty, racism, sexism, ableism, adultism, and other forms of oppression, they are often blamed and held responsible for their difficulties, i.e. blaming the victim (Amala, 2012; Kriegler & Bester, 2014; McGibbon, 2012). Moreover, the very existence of the mental health system in its current form deliberately diverts attention away from taking action to liberate humans from societal oppression, and instead focuses on labelling, pathologizing, and medicating responses to trauma and oppression. Problems such as racial profiling, poverty, domestic violence, homophobia, and exclusion of people with disabilities are viciously framed as personal defects rather than societal failures (Amala, 2012; Kriegler & Bester, 2014; McGibbon, 2012).

Adding insult to injury, once someone receives a psychiatric label – another oppression takes hold. People are stigmatized with a psychiatric label, and they then begin to self-stigmatize – believing there is something inherently wrong with them (Corrigan et al., 2006). Psychiatric drugs are often the first line of intervention. Although these drugs are experienced as helpful by many, they also have a host of negative side effects including increased suicidal ideation, decreased libido, cognitive decline, cardiac complications, metabolic syndrome, tardive dyskinesia, kidney problems, as well as tolerance and dependence (Moncrieff et al., 2013). Some of these side effects contribute to the 10–25-year reduction in life span of people labelled with serious mental illness who are disproportionately affected by cardiovascular, respiratory, and infectious diseases, diabetes, hypertension, and suicide (WHO, 2013).

A recent emphasis on trauma-informed care (TIC) in the mental health field and anti-oppressive practice (AOP), a particular social work model, is transforming the mental health system away from the medicalization of mental anguish towards a humane and relational approach to addressing developmental, historical, and current trauma (Curry-Stevens, 2012; Levenson, 2017; Substance Abuse and Mental Health Services Administration, 2014; Sweeney et al., 2018). Within these approaches, instead of seeking to understand what is wrong with our clients, a pivotal focus becomes understanding what happened to our clients.

In the context of the pandemic, many oppressed groups are experiencing increased targeting, and those with and without psychiatric labels are experiencing both increased trauma or re-triggering of early trauma. Disruptions in daily occupations, combined with the devastating loss of loved ones and the loss of economic security place many people at increased risk for severe mental distress and substance use. Despite the challenges confronting humanity in the pandemic, every human has the capacity to heal, recover, and re-emerge from trauma and oppression. Whether through peer support or professional services, individual or group work, community organizing or activism, religion and spirituality or the creation of art, collaborative reparations of the planet, or caring for sick and vulnerable humans, a focus on healing is essential. Infusing compassionate listening and supporting the release of emotional distress through tears, laughter, shaking, and talking is fundamental to recovery and re-emergence from both current trauma and triggering of past trauma.

Older people: Bold elders

Ageism, or the stereotyping, prejudice, and discrimination towards people on the basis of age, stems from the perception that people might be too old "to be" or "to do something" (Officer & de la Fuente-Núñez (2019). While ageism is just as pervasive as more blatant forms of discrimination such as sexism and racism, it remains largely unrecognized and unchallenged (Officer & de la Fuente-Núñez, 2019). In other words, the association between ageing and declining physical and mental abilities are subtly and not so subtly embedded in structures within society and harmfully situated in our minds as we devalue older people. This is tragically evident in the pandemic which not only kills those over 80 at a rate five times higher than the global average, but also places older people at a greater risk of discrimination when it comes to scarce medical resources (UN News, 2020).

Pascoe and Richman's important meta-analysis of 134 studies highlights the significant negative effect that perceived discrimination has on both physical and mental health (2009). Levy et al. (2012) found that older adults with negative age stereotypes were less likely to recover from severe disability as measured by participation in activities of daily living (bathing, dressing, transferring, and walking) than people with positive age stereotypes. Furthermore, people with negative stereotypes about ageing live an average of 7.5 years less than those who hold positive attitudes (Levy et al., 2002). These data raise an alarm regarding the potential health consequences of internalizing the pandemic's amplified negative messaging about one's value as an older person. Fortunately, United Nations Secretary-General António Guterres is countering the current rise in discrimination towards older people by reminding us that older people contribute "immeasurably" to their families and communities, and "No person, young or old, is expendable" (UN News, 2020, p. 1).

While some cultural groups, such as South Korean, Native American, Greek, and Chinese people are thought of as holding elders in high regard, research on cultural differences in attitudes towards older people is inconsistent. Zhang et al. (2016) found that although personal communal values such as friendliness, warmth, and love are positively correlated with positive attitudes towards older adults, cultural values might not be as robust in influencing attitudes towards older adults as previously thought. However, using Kogan's Attitudes toward Old People scale, Morrisseau et al. (2017) found that Indigenous Canadians, both male and female, and those living on and off reservations, had positive attitudes towards their elders and a relatively more positive attitude compared with an undergraduate sample of mostly Caucasian individuals.

Pacific Islanders and Pilipino/a heritage people: Caring, unified, and compassionate

Pacific Islanders and Pilipino heritage people are Indigenous people who live on the islands that extend from the south of Japan to Southeast Asia, to the South Pacific, and Aotearoa (New Zealand). They have resisted oppression and the theft of their resources for centuries and held onto their distinct "island cultures". Yet the effects of colonization have multiple, ongoing negative health consequences for people of the Pacific. For example, forced abandonment of their traditional diet has resulted in a high prevalence of obesity and related health problems (WHO, 2010). In some Pacific Island nations, more than 50%, and in some cases up to 90%, of the population is overweight (WHO, 2010). Under colonial rule, importation of food became the norm, and traditional food growing and preparation practices were lost (McLennan & Ulijaszek, 2014).

Many Pacific Island nations have managed to keep the coronavirus at bay – perhaps due to their geographic isolation, swift action to practise social distancing, and banning travel to and from these nations early in the pandemic (Welle, 2020). In the United States, Hawaii is successfully limiting the spread of the virus, yet Native Hawaiian and Pacific Islander residents in other states report a higher rate of COVID-19 infection than any other racial or cultural group in the United States (Kaholokula et al., 2020). The health consequences of long-standing poverty are implicated in these alarming rates of COVID-19 (Kaholokula et al., 2020).

Sex trafficking is a heinous injustice experienced by women and children across the globe. A report on sexual exploitation of children in travel and tourism in the Pacific region suggests the increasing vulnerability of precious Pacific Island children to this deplorable industry as tourism grows within broken economies (Presquer, 2016). The First World Congress Against Commercial Sexual Exploitation of Children was held in Stockholm in 1996. Although some progress has been made across the globe in protecting children from the devastating and damaging experience of sex trafficking, greater resources must be dedicated to ending all forms of sexual exploitation. The magnificent values and practices of Native Hawaiian and Pacific Island people, aloha (compassion), mālama (caring), and lōkahi (unity), said differently across cultural groups, guide them in overcoming any challenge

(Kaholokula, et al., 2020). Given the many cultural strengths of Pacific Islanders, eliminating sexual exploitation is fully within their power.

Parents: Mothers and fathers as shapers of a loving world

Parents are not thought of as an oppressed group, but are seen as both the key nurturers and sometimes the key agents of oppression towards their children. The work of parenting is some of the most important and complex work in the world. With over 100 billion nerve cells, there is nothing more complex than the human mind, and the true flourishing of a developing mind requires a great deal of thought and loving attention from parents, an extended family, a community, and society. Rather than treating the work of parenting as a central and key occupation within modern societies, the work of parenting is treated more like a hobby – something done in addition to another, more important job (Wipfler & Schore, 2016). The working conditions of most parents, the primary caregivers of children, are abysmal. Although there are a growing number of initiatives to recognize and support the work of parenting in Scandinavian countries and beyond, parents generally receive no training, no pay for their 24/7 work, no breaks, and no emotional support. What they do receive is a great deal of blame and criticism for any difficulties their children exhibit throughout their life course. Just as men can be viewed as oppressed by society and the social construct of masculinity, parents can also be viewed as oppressed by societal structures that do not value children, the work of parenting, and families.

A recent study found that stress associated with adjustment to parenthood during the first year has a worse impact on a person's life satisfaction than divorce, unemployment, and even the death of a partner (Cha, 2015; Margolis & Myrskylä, 2015). Rachel Margolis and Mikko Myrskylä (2015) followed more than 2,000 Germans from being childless until 2 years after the birth of their first child. Although about 30% remained in the same state of happiness or better once their child was born, 70% indicated that their happiness decreased during the first and second years after their child was born. The average drop in happiness, 1.4 units, was considered severe (Margolis & Myrskylä, 2015). By comparison, other studies have quantified the impact of other major life events on the same happiness scale and found that divorce had the equivalent of a 0.6 "happiness unit" drop; unemployment had a 1.0 unit drop; and the death of a partner had a 1.0 unit drop (Cha, 2015). Margolis and Myrskylä (2015) found that the drop in wellbeing surrounding the birth of a first child is a strong predictor of whether or not parents will have a second child. According to the World Population Review (2019), nations with the lowest fertility rates (each below 1.25) are South Korea, Taiwan, Macau, Singapore, and Puerto Rico. Few parents in these nations are choosing to have more than one child – perhaps due to the oppression of parents.

The oppression of parents has perhaps never been more evident than in the pandemic. A sizeable number of parents are now called upon to simultaneously engage in paid work at home while doing the essential work of parenting. Many parents in the United States report that although they feel closeness and warmth with their children, financial concerns and social isolation are interfering with their ability to parent (Lee & Ward, 2020). Under duress, they are yelling, screaming, and physically disciplining their children more often than prior to the pandemic (Lee & Ward, 2020).

People with disabilities: Elegant and essential humans

According to WHO (2018), about 15% of the world's population has some form of disability, and rates of disability are on the rise due to an ageing population and increases in chronic health conditions. Accessing health care is a significant problem for many people with disabilities due to cost, limited availability, physical barriers, and inadequate skills on the part of health practitioners (WHO, 2018). Additionally, living with a disability is often stressful and isolating, and both factors may have a negative impact on health and health behaviours such as smoking, substance use, and risk-taking behaviours, nutrition, and physical activity (Turk & McDermott, 2018). Macdonald et al. (2018) compared experiences of able-bodied people and people with disabilities in the UK and found that people with disabilities were significantly overrepresented among the population who are lonely and isolated, and those with learning impairments reported the highest feelings of isolation and loneliness. Sadly, 61% of participants with disabilities acknowledged that they spent most of their time alone, compared with 28% of the group without disabilities; and 71% agreed they would like more contact, compared with 46% of the non-disabled group. Environmental barriers were a key problem. Holt-Lunstad et al. (2017) cite a robust body of scientific evidence indicating that having many high-quality close relationships and feeling socially connected is associated with a decreased risk for all-cause mortality as well as a range of diseases, and advocate for advancing social connection as a public health priority.

According to the CDC (2020), people with disabilities are not inherently at greater risk of becoming infected with or seriously ill from COVID-19. However, underlying medical conditions such as lung disease, heart conditions, or a weakened immune system may make them vulnerable to the virus. The limitations on mobility that make social distancing challenging, a difficulty in understanding and practising preventative measures, and the difficulty of communicating symptoms of the illness can also place some people with disabilities at great risk.

Poor/working-class people: Proud and brilliant world changers

In 2011, Pew researchers estimated that 71% of the world's people were on a low income or poor, living on $10 or less a day (Kochar, 2015). Although those earning $10.01 to $20.00 per day, or 13% of the global population, were considered middle class, others might define these workers as working class. Regardless of the often-blurred lines between working- and middle-class people, poor, working-class, and some middle-class people are the producers of goods and services that global economies depend upon. They include farmers, construction/manufacturing workers, health care workers, sanitation workers, housekeepers, store clerks, teachers, artists, secretaries, transportation workers, janitors, cooks, cashiers, servers, office/technical support workers and more. Despite their inherent value as humans and the essential nature of their work, far too many poor, working-class, and some middle-class people and families across the globe struggle to exist on their wages. In the pandemic, many of the essential workers in the United States and throughout the world who are risking their lives for the wellbeing of all are working-class and poor people (Theoharis, 2020).

With a few exceptions, a history of colonization is the number one reason for poverty among nations of the world followed by war and political instability, debt to wealthy nations, discrimination and social inequality, and vulnerability to a natural disaster (Williams, 2016). Despite a decline in extreme poverty over recent years, about half of the world's population or 3.4 billion people, are living on less than $5.50 a day and are unable to meet their basic human needs (World Bank, 2018). World Bank projections estimate that COVID-19 is likely to cause an increase in global poverty for the first time since 1998 – pushing an additional 40–60 million people into extreme poverty in 2020. Sub-Saharan Africa might be hit the hardest (Mahler et al., 2020). Poverty is the major enemy of health in economically poor nations (developing world) because it forces large numbers of people to live without decent shelter, clean water, or adequate sanitation (WHO, 2019b). Additionally, half the world lacks access to essential health services (WHO, 2017).

In the United States, inequality and poverty were destroying many lives before COVID-19 arrived (Theoharis, 2020). More than 38 million people in the United States were living below the federal poverty line (Semega et al., 2019). Yet the federal poverty line, established in 1964, doesn't take into account household expenses that have been common to Americans for decades – health care, child care, housing, and transportation (Theoharis, 2020). The Poor People's Campaign and the Institute for Policy Studies, using the Census Bureau's Supplemental Poverty Measure as a baseline, estimates that there were actually at least 140 million people in the United States who were poor – "or just a $400 emergency away from that state" prior to COVID-19 (Theoharis, 2020, n.p.). Many lacked health insurance and could not afford to nurture themselves and their families with the kind of food and living environments that sustain health. In fact, a comparison of the most affluent 1% with the poorest 1% across racial groups in the United States found a life expectancy gap of 15 years less for poor men and 10 years less for poor women (Chetty et al., 2016). One's zip code in the United States was found to be a predictor of poverty and racial discrimination, and an indicator of how long people live (California Endowment, 2015).

Young people and young adults: A powerful and key force for change

DeJong and Love (2015) conceptualize young people, those ranging in age from young children to young adults, as occupying a subordinate status in society. In a sense, every person has experienced oppression in that all young people across the world are mistreated and disrespected by adults simply for being young people (DeJong & Love, 2013).

The Adverse Childhood Experiences Study (ACE Study) exposed the harsh reality of adversity that many young people endure during sensitive developmental years (Felitti et al., 1998). Categories of childhood experiences studied included psychological, physical, or sexual abuse; violence against mother; or living with household members who were substance abusers, mentally ill or suicidal, or ever imprisoned. More than half of the respondents reported at least one adverse childhood experience (ACE) and one-fourth reported two or more ACEs. A strong relationship was found between the number of ACEs and adult diseases including ischaemic heart disease, cancer, chronic lung disease, skeletal fractures, and liver disease. People who had experienced four or more categories of childhood exposure, compared to those who had experienced none, had a 4- to 12-fold increased health risk for alcoholism, drug abuse, depression, and suicide attempt. They also experienced a 2- to 4-fold increase in smoking, poor self- rated health, ≥ 50 sexual intercourse partners, and sexually transmitted diseases. They had a 1.4- to 1.6-fold increase in physical inactivity and severe obesity.

In a recent analysis, almost half of children in the United States were found to have experienced one ACE, and sadly, the most common ACEs reported were economic hardship (particularly among rural children) and the divorce or separation of a parent or guardian (Crouch et al., 2019). Placing them at high risk for chronic health and social problems, one in ten children were found to have experienced three or more ACEs. Racism's life-altering tentacles have a devastating impact on children as evidenced in ACE numbers showing that 61% of Black non-Hispanic children, 51% of Hispanic children, 40% of white non-Hispanic children, and 23% of Asian children were found to have experienced at least one ACE (Crouch et al., 2019).

As Lee and Ward (2020) noted, children in the pandemic are experiencing both greater contact and affection from parents, yet also more verbal and physical abuse than previously. Poverty is worsening for many children across the globe, and the loss of educational opportunities due to school closures may have lasting negative social and health consequences (Lancker & Parolin, 2020). Effective collaborative leadership from multiple stakeholders across racial and cultural lines is needed to develop communities that support the flourishing of all families and children.

REFERENCES

Ahn, M. (2020, April 13). Combating COVID–19: Lessons from South Korea. Brookings: TechTank. www.brookings.edu/blog/techtank/2020/04/13/combating-covid-19-lessons-from-south-korea/

Amala, O. (2020, October 30). Mental health and social oppression: Seeing the connection. LSE: The London School of Economics and Political Science. Blog post. https://blogs.lse.ac.uk/equityDiversityInclusion/2012/10/mental-health-and-social-oppression-seeing-the-connection/

American Cancer Society (2019). *Cancer facts and figures for African Americans.* www.cancer.org/content/dam/cancer-org/research/cancer-facts-and-statistics/cancer-facts-and-figures-for-african-americans/cancer-facts-and-figures-for-african-americans-2019-2021.pdf

American Psychological Association (2017, August 3). Fat shaming in the doctor's office can be mentally and physically harmful: Health care providers may offer weight loss advice in place of medical treatment, researchers say. ScienceDaily. www.sciencedaily.com/releases/2017/08/170803092015.htm

Ammar, N., Couture-Carron, A., Alvi, S., & San Antonio, J. (2013, December). Experiences of Muslim and non-Muslim battered immigrant women with the police in the U.S.: A closer understanding of commonalities and differences. *Violence Against Women, 19*(12), 1449–1471. https://doi.org/10.1177/1077801213517565

Bada, F. (2018). The poorest countries in Asia. GraphicMaps. www.graphicmaps.com/the-poorest-countries-in-asia

Baker, P., Dworkin, S. L., Tong, S., Banks, I., Shand, T., & Yamey, G. (2014). The men's health gap: Men must be included in the global health equity agenda. *Bulletin of the World Health Organization, 92*, 618–620. http://dx.doi.org/10.2471/BLT.13.132795

Bernstein, H., Gonzalez, D., Karpman, M., & Zuckerman, S. (2019, May 22). One in seven adults in immigrant families reported avoiding public benefit programs in 2018. Urban Institute. www.urban.org/sites/default/files/publication/100270/one_in_seven_adults_in_immigrant_families_reported_avoiding_publi_7.pdf

Black Women's Roundtable (2015, March 26). *Black women in the United States: 2015.* www.ncbcp.org/news/releases/BWRReport.BlackWomeninU.S.2015.3.26.15FINAL.pdf

Boucher, N. (2017, May 19). Supporting Muslim patients during advanced stages of illness. *The Permanente Journal, 21*,16–190. https://doi.org/10.7812/tpp/16-190

Burki, T. (2020, April 17). COVID-19 in Latin America. *The Lancet: Infectious Diseases, 20*(5), 511–628. https://doi:10.1016/S1473-3099(20)30303-0

California Endowment (2015, October 6). Your zip code says a lot about your health. www.calendow.org/news/your-zip-code-says-a-lot-about-your-health/

Carr, E. R., Szymanski, D. M., Taha, F., West, L. M., & Kaslow, N. J. (2014). Understanding the link between multiple oppressions and depression among African American women: The role of internalization. *Psychology of Women Quarterly, 38*(2), 233–245. https://doi.org/10.1177/0361684313499900

Centers for Disease Control and Prevention (CDC) (2019). Heart disease facts. www.cdc.gov/heartdisease/facts.htm

Centers for Disease Control and Prevention (CDC) (2020). Coronavirus disease 2019 (COVID-19): People with disabilities. www.cdc.gov/coronavirus/2019-ncov/need-extra-precautions/people-with-disabilities.html

Cha, A. E. (2015, August 11). It turns out parenthood is worse than divorce, unemployment – even the death of a partner. *The Washington Post.* Blog post. www.washingtonpost.com/news/to-your-health/wp/2015/08/11/the-most-depressing-statistic-imaginable-about-being-a-new-parent/&xid=17259,1500000,15700022,15700124,15700149,15700168,15700173,15700186,15700201

Chelala, C. (2019, March 21). Public health challenges in Latin America and the Caribbean. CounterPunch. www.counterpunch.org/2019/03/21/public-health-challenges-in-latin-america-and-the-caribbean/

Chetty, R., Stepner, M., Abraham, S., Lin, S., Scuderi, B., Turner, N., … Cutler, D. (2016, April 26). The association between income and life expectancy in the U.S., 2001–2014. *Journal of the American Medical Association, 315*(16), 1750–1766. https://doi.org/10.1001/jama.2016.4226

Chotner, I. (2019, July 13). How the stress of separation and detention changes the lives of children. *The New Yorker.* www.newyorker.com/news/q-and-a/how-the-stress-of-separation-and-detention-changes-the-lives-of-children

Connell, T. (2020, April 13). Migrant workers essential workers not only in COVID-19. Solidarity Center: AFL-CIO. www.solidaritycenter.org/migrant-workers-essential-workers-not-only-in-covid-19/

Corley, J. (2020, April 21). Why refugees are the world's most vulnerable people during the COVID-19 pandemic. *Forbes.* www.forbes.com/sites/jacquelyncorley/2020/04/21/why-refugees-are-the-worlds-most-vulnerable-people-during-the-covid-19-pandemic/#3b1dec874112

Corrigan, R. C., Watson, A. C., & Barr, L. (2006). The self-stigma of mental illness: Implications for self-esteem and self-efficacy. *Journal of Social and Clinical Psychology, 25*(8), 875–884. https://doi.org/10.1521/jscp.2006.25.8.875

Crouch, E., Probst, J. P., Radcliff, E., Bennett, K. J., & McKinney, S. H. (2019, June). Prevalence of adverse childhood experiences (ACEs) among US children. *Child Abuse and Neglect, 92*, 209–2018. https://doi:10.1016/j.chiabu.2019.04.010

Curry-Stevens, A. C. (2012). Persuasion: Infusing advocacy practice with insights from anti-oppression practice. *Journal of Social Work, 12*(4), 345–363. https://doi.org/10.1177/1468017310387252

DeJong, K., & Love, B. (2013). Ageism and adultism. In M. Adams, W. J. Blumenfeld, R. Castañeda, H. Hackman, M. Peters & X. Zúñiga (Eds), *Readings for diversity and social justice* (3rd ed., pp. 470–474). New York: Routledge.

DeJong, K., & Love, B. J. (2015). Youth oppression as a technology of colonialism: Conceptual frameworks and possibilities for social justice education. *Praxis, Equity & Excellence in Education, 48*(3), 489–508. https://doi.org/10.1080/10665684.2015.1057086

Desjardins, B. (2004). Why is life expectancy longer for women than it is for men? *Scientific American, 291*(6), 120–120. www.scientificamerican.com/article/why-is-life-expectancy-lo/

Edwards, F., Lee, H., & Esposito, M. (2019, August 20). Risk of being killed by police use of force in the United States by age, race, ethnicity, and sex. *Proceedings of the National Academy of Sciences of the United States of America, 116*(34), 16793–16798. https://doi.org/10.1073/pnas.1821204116

Felitti, V. J., Anda, R. F., Nordenberg, D., & Williamson, D. F. (1998). Adverse childhood experiences and health outcomes in adults: The ACE study. *Journal of Family and Consumer Sciences, 90*(3), 31.

Flores, A. (2017, September 18). How the U.S. Hispanic population is changing. Pew Research Center. www.pewresearch.org/fact-tank/2017/09/18/how-the-u-s-hispanic-population-is-changing/

Global Forum (2017, July). *Agenda 2030 for LGBTI health and wellbeing.* https://msmgf.org/wp-content/uploads/2017/07/Agenda-2030-for-LGBTI-Health_July-2017.pdf

Goodney, P. P., Dzebisashvil, N., Goodman, D. C., & Bronner, K. K. (2013). *Variation in the care of surgical conditions: Diabetes and peripheral arterial disease.* Lebanon, NH: The Dartmouth Institute for Health Policy and Clinical Practice. www.diabetesincontrol.com/wp-content/uploads/2014/10/www.dartmouthatlas.org_downloads_reports_Diabetes_report_10_14_14.pdf

Guttentag, L., & Driscoll, S. (2019, April 22). Crisis at the border? An update on immigration policy with Stanford's Lucas Guttentag. SLS Blogs. https://law.stanford.edu/2019/04/22/crisis-at-the-border-an-update-on-immigration-policy-with-stanfords-lucas-guttentag/

Hall, G., & Gandolfo, A. (2016, August 9). Poverty and exclusion among Indigenous peoples: The global experience. World Bank Blogs. https://blogs.worldbank.org/voices/poverty-and-exclusion-among-indigenous-peoples-global-evidence

Halter, M. J., & Varcarolis, E. M. (2014). *Varcarolis' foundations of psychiatric mental health nursing: A clinical approach* (7th ed.). St Louis, MO: Elsevier/Saunders.

Hamel, K., Tong, B., & Hofer, M. (2019, March 28). Poverty in Africa is now falling – but not fast enough. Brookings. www.brookings.edu/blog/future-development/2019/03/28/poverty-in-africa-is-now-falling-but-not-fast-enough/

Hammonds, E. M., & Reverby, S. M. (2019, September 4). Toward a historically informed analysis of racial health disparities since 1619. *American Journal of Public Health.* https://ajph.aphapublications.org/doi/10.2105/AJPH.2019.305262

Health Poverty Action (2018). Women and girls: Women and girls are disproportionately impacted by poverty. www.healthpovertyaction.org/how-poverty-is-created/women-girls/

Herrera, J. (2019). Most terrorist victims are Muslim. *Pacific Standard.* https://psmag.com/news/most-terrorist-victims-are-muslim

Holt-Lunstad, J., Robles, T. F., & Sbarra, D. A. (2017). Advancing social connection as a public health priority in the U.S. *The American Psychologist, 72*(6), 517–530. https://doi.org/10.1037/amp0000103

Hutson, D. J. (2017). Teaching critical perspectives on body weight: The obesity "epidemic" and pro-ana movement in classroom discussions. *Teaching Sociology, 45*(1), 41–53. https://doi.org/10.1177/0092055x16664396

Kaholokula, J. K., Samoa, R., Miyamoto, R. E. S., Palafox, N., & Daniels, S. (2020, May). COVID-19 special column: COVID-19 hits native Hawaiian and Pacific Islander communities the hardest. *Hawai'i Journal of Health & Social Welfare*, *79*(5), 143–146. https://hawaiijournalhealth.org/past_issues/HJHSW_May20.pdf

Kass, D. A., Duggal, P., & Cingolani, A. (2020, May 4). Obesity could shift severe COVID-19 disease to younger ages. *The Lancet*. www.thelancet.com/journals/lancet/article/PIIS0140-6736(20)31024-2/fulltext

Kasstan, B. (2020, April 16). Opinion: Angry at ultra-Orthodox Jews for 'defying' coronavirus rules? It's more complicated than that. Haaretz. www.haaretz.com/world-news/.premium-angry-at-ultra-orthodox-jews-for-defying-covid-19-rules-it-s-more-complicated-1.8764711

Kochar, R. (2015, July 8). A global middle class is more promise than reality. Pew Research Center. www.pewresearch.org/global/2015/07/08/a-global-middle-class-is-more-promise-than-reality/

Kriegler, S., & Bester, S. E. (2014, November 25). A critical engagement with the DSM-5 and psychiatric diagnosis. *Journal of Psychology in Africa*, *24*(4), 393–401. https://doi.org/10.1080/14330237.2014.980629

Lancker, W. V., & Parolin, Z. (2020, April 7). COVID-19, school closures, and child poverty: A social crisis in the making. *Lancet: Public Health*. https://doi.org/10.1016/S2468-2667(20)30084-0

Lavers, M. K. (2020, April 27). Countries urged to stop targeting LGBTQ people during coronavirus pandemic. Washington Blade: America's LGBT News Source. www.washingtonblade.com/2020/04/27/countries-urged-to-stop-targeting-lgbtq-people-during-coronavirus-pandemic/

Leavitt, R. A., Ertl, A., Sheats, K., Petrosky, E., Ivey-Stephenson, A., & Fowler, K. A. (2018). Suicides among American Indian/Alaska Natives: National Violent Death Reporting System, 18 States, 2003–2014. *Centers for Disease Control and Prevention – Morbidity and Mortality Weekly Report*, *67*(8), 237–242. doi: 10.15585/mmwr.mm6708a1

Lee, S. J., & Ward, K. P. (2020, March 26). Research brief: Stress and parenting during the coronavirus pandemic. Parenting in Context: Research Lab. www.parentingincontext.org/uploads/8/1/3/1/81318622/research_brief_stress_and_parenting_during_the_coronavirus_pandemic_final.pdf

Legatum Institute (2018). *Legatum prosperity index 2018* (12th ed.). https://prosperitysite.s3-accelerate.amazonaws.com/2515/4321/8072/2018_Prosperity_Index.pdf

Levenson, J. (2017, April). Trauma-informed social work practice. *Social Work*, *62*(2), 105–113. https://doi.org/10.1093/sw/swx001

Levy, B. R., Slade, M. D., Kunkel, S. R., & Kasl, S. V. (2002). Longevity increased by positive self-perceptions of aging. *Journal of Personality and Social Psychology*, *83*(2), 261.

Levy, B. R., Slade, M. D., Murphy, T. E., & Gill, T. M. (2012). Association between positive age stereotypes and recovery from disability in older persons. *Journal of the American Medical Association*, *308*(19), 1972. https://doi.org/10.1001/jama.2012.14541

Lewis, J. F., Zeger, S. L., Li, X., Mann, N. C., Newgard, C. D., Haynes, S., … McCarthy, M. L. (2019). Gender differences in the quality of EMS care nationwide for chest pain and out-of-hospital cardiac arrest. *Women's Health Issues*, *29*(2), 116–124. https://doi.org/10.1016/j.whi.2018.10.007

Lipka, M. (2017, August 9). Muslims and Islam: Key findings in the U.S. and around the world. Pew Research Center. www.pewresearch.org/fact-tank/2017/08/09/muslims-and-islam-key-findings-in-the-u-s-and-around-the-world/

Loewenthal, K. M. (2012). Mental health and mental health care for Jews in the diaspora, with particular reference to the UK. *The Israel Journal of Psychiatry and Related Sciences*, *49*(3), 159–166.

Loffman, M. (2020, April 7). Asian Americans describe 'gut punch' of racist attacks during coronavirus pandemic. PBS News Hour. www.pbs.org/newshour/nation/asian-americans-describe-gut-punch-of-racist-attacks-during-coronavirus-pandemic

Macdonald, S. J., Deacon, L., Nixon, J., Akintola, A., Gillingham, A., Kent, J., ... Highmore, L. (2018). 'The invisible enemy': Disability, loneliness and isolation. *Disability & Society*, *33*(7), 1138–1159. https://doi:10.1080/09687599.2018.1476224

Mahler, D. G., Lakner, C., Aguilar, A.C., & Wu, H. (2020). The impact of COVID-19 (Coronavirus) on global poverty: Why Sub–Saharan Africa might be the region hardest hit. World Bank Blogs. https://blogs.worldbank.org/opendata/impact-covid-19-coronavirus-global-poverty-why-sub-saharan-africa-might-be-region-hardest

Margolis, R., & Myrskylä, M. (2015). Parental well-being surrounding first birth as a determinant of further parity progression. *Demography*, *52*(4), 1147–1166. https://doi:10.1007/s13524-015-0413-2

McLennan, A. K., & Ulijaszek, S. J. (2014). Obesity emergence in the Pacific islands: Why understanding colonial history and social change is important. *Public Health Nutrition*, *18*(8), 1499–1505. https://doi:10.1017/s136898001400175x

McGibbon, E. (2012). *Oppression: A social determinant of health*. Black Point, Nova Scotia: Fernwood Publishing.

Mihtra, M. (2018). Eight important facts about poverty in Asia. The Borgen Project. Blog post. https://borgenproject.org/causes-of-poverty-in-asia/

Mogahed, D., & Chouhoud, Y. (2017). American Muslim poll 2017: Muslims at the crossroads. Institute for Social Policy and Understanding. www.ispu.org/wp-content/uploads/2017/03/American-Muslim-Poll-2017-Report.pdf

Moncrieff, J., Cohen, D., & Porter, S. (2013, November). The psychoactive effects of psychiatric medicine: The elephant in the room. *Journal of Psychoactive Drugs*, *45*(5), 409–415. www.ncbi.nlm.nih.gov/pmc/articles/PMC4118946/

Morrisseau, N. R., Caswell, J. M., Sinclair, A., & Valliant, P. M. (2017). Indigenous Peoples' attitude toward their elders and associated personality correlates. SAGE Open. https://doi.org/10.1177/2158244017697166

Nasim, I. (2020, April 29). Patience, sacrifice and Zakat: How Muslims find the strength to endure the COVID-19 pandemic. Euronews. www.euronews.com/2020/04/29/patience-sacrifice-zakat-how-muslims-find-the-strength-to-endure-covid-19-pandemic-view

National Institute on Minority Health and Health Disparities (2016). The Center for Asian health engages communities in research to reduce Asian American health disparities. www.nimhd.nih.gov/news-events/features/training-workforce-dev/center-asian-health.html

New, C. (2001). Oppressed and oppressors? The systematic mistreatment of men. *Sociology*, *35*(3), 729–748. https://doi.org/10.1177/S0038038501000372

Nuwer, R. (2020, May 4). The indigenous communities that predicted Covid-19. BBC: Travel. www.bbc.com/travel/story/20200503-the-indigenous-communities-that-predicted-covid-19

Office of the Surgeon General and National Action Alliance for Suicide Prevention (2012, September). *2012 National strategy for suicide prevention: Goals and objectives for action*. U.S. Department of Health and Human Services, Substance Abuse and Mental Health Services Administration. www.ncbi.nlm.nih.gov/books/NBK109917/

Officer, A., & de la Fuente-Núñez, V. (2018). A global campaign to combat ageism. *Bulletin of the World Health Organization, 96*(4), 295. www.ncbi.nlm.nih.gov/pmc/articles/PMC5872010/

Ostler, J. (2020, April 29). Disease has never been just disease for Native Americans. *Atlantic.* www.theatlantic.com/ideas/archive/2020/04/disease-has-never-been-just-disease-native-americans/610852/

Pascoe, E. A., & Richman, L. S. (2009). Perceived discrimination and health: A meta-analytic review. *Psychological Bulletin, 135*(4), 531–554. https://doi:10.1037/a0016059

Poupart, L. M. (2003). The familiar face of genocide: Internalized oppression among American Indians. *Hypatia, 18*(2), 86–100. www.webpages.uidaho.edu/engl484jj/18.2poupart.pdf

Presquer, C. (2016). *Global study on sexual exploitation of children in travel and tourism: Regional Report: Pacific: 2016.* ECPAT International jointly with Defence for Children. www.protectingchildrenintourism.org/wp-content/uploads/2018/05/PACIFIC-Region.pdf

Puhl, R. M., Andreyeva, T., & Brownell, K. D. (2008). Perceptions of weight discrimination: Prevalence and comparison to race and gender discrimination in America. *International Journal of Obesity, 32*(6), 992. https://doi:10.1038/ijo.2008.22

Puhl, R. M., & Heuer, C. A. (2009). The stigma of obesity: a review and update. *Obesity, 17*(5), 941–964.

Regan, J. C., & Partridge, L. (2013). Gender and longevity: Why do men die earlier than women? Comparative and experimental evidence. *Best Practice & Research: Clinical Endocrinology & Metabolism, 27*(4), 467–479. http://doi:10.1016/j.beem.2013.05.016

Representation Project, The (2019). *The mask you live in: The boy crisis in America.* http://therepresentationproject.org/film/the-mask-you-live-in-film/the-issue/

Rescue.org (2018, June). Migrants, asylum seekers, refugees and immigrants: What's the difference? International Rescue Committee. www.rescue.org/article/migrants-asylum-seekers-refugees-and-immigrants-whats-difference

Semega, J., Kollar, M., Creamer, J., & Mohanty, A. (2019, September 10). Income and poverty in the United States: 2018. United States Census Bureau. www.census.gov/library/publications/2019/demo/p60-266.html

Shaver, J., Sharma, A., & Stephenson, R. (2018). Rural primary care providers' experiences and knowledge regarding LGBTQ health in a midwestern state. *The Journal of Rural Health, 35*(3), 362–373. http://doi:10.1111/jrh.12322

Shetty, S. (2019). Most dangerous journey: What Central American migrants face when they try to cross the border. Amnesty International. www.amnestyusa.org/most-dangerous-journey-what-central-american-migrants-face-when-they-try-to-cross-the-border/

Singh, M., & Jirabm, N. (2020, April 18). 'The virus doesn't discriminate but governments do': Latinos disproportionately hit by coronavirus. The Guardian. www.theguardian.com/us-news/2020/apr/18/the-virus-doesnt-discriminate-but-governments-do-latinos-disproportionately-hit-by-coronavirus

Skodo, A. (2017, April 22). How immigration detention compares around the world. The Conversation. https://theconversation.com/how-immigration-detention-compares-around-the-world-76067

Sternlicht, A. (2020, May 19). Navajo nation has most coronavirus infections per capita in the U.S., beating New York, New Jersey. *Forbes.* www.forbes.com/sites/alexandrasternlicht/2020/05/19/navajo-nation-has-most-coronavirus-infections-per-capita-in-us-beating-new-york-new-jersey/#4fa6ea768b10

Substance Abuse and Mental Health Services Administration (2014). *SAMHSA's concept of trauma and guidance for a trauma-informed approach*. HHS Publication No. (SMA) 14–4884. https://ncsacw.samhsa.gov/userfiles/files/SAMHSA_Trauma.pdf

Sweeney, A., Filson, B., Kennedy, A., Collinson, L., & Gillard, S. (2018, September). A paradigm shift: Relationships in trauma-informed mental health services. *British Journal of Psychiatry Advances*, *24*(5), 319–333. www.ncbi.nlm.nih.gov/pmc/articles/PMC6088388/

Theoharis, L. (2020, April 22). Inequality and poverty were destroying America well before Covid-19. *The Nation*. www.thenation.com/article/society/inequality-and-poverty-were-destroying-america-well-before-covid-19/

Tian, Q., Wang, A., Zuo, Y., Chen, S., Hou, H., Wang, W., ... & Wang, Y. (2020). All-cause mortality in metabolically healthy individuals was not predicted by overweight and obesity. JCI insight, 5(16). doi: 10.1172/jci.insight.136982

Toomey, R. B., Syvertsen, A. K., & Shramko, M. (2018). Transgender adolescent suicide behavior. *Pediatrics*, *142*(4), e20174218. http://doi:10.1542/peds.2017-4218

Touchin, J. (2020, May 18). 69 new cases of COVID-19, two more deaths and 928 recoveries reported. Press release. The Navajo Nation – Office of the President and Vice President. www.navajo-nsn.gov/News%20Releases/OPVP/2020/May/FOR%20IMMEDIATE%20RELEASE%20-%2069%20new%20cases%20of%20COVID-19_%20two%20more%20deaths%20and%20928%20recoveries%20reported.pdf

Turk, M. A., & McDermott, S. (2018). Disability, stress, and health disparities. *Disability and Health Journal*, *11*(3), 331–332. doi: 10.1016/j.dhjo.2018.05.001

UNHCR (2018). *Desperate journeys: Executive summary*. www.unhcr.org/desperatejourneys/#foreword

United Nations (UN) (2020, April 9). Policy brief: The impact of COVID-19 on women. www.unwomen.org/-/media/headquarters/attachments/sections/library/publications/2020/policy-brief-the-impact-of-covid-19-on-women-en.pdf?la=en&vs=1406

UN News (2020, May 1). 'Rights and dignity' of older people must be respected during COVID-19 and beyond. https://news.un.org/en/story/2020/05/1063052

UN Women (2020, March 9). Opening statement by Under-Secretary-General of the United Nations and Executive Director of UN Women, Phumzile Mlambo-Ngcuka, at the 64th session of the Commission on the Status of Women 9 March 2020. www.unwomen.org/en/news/stories/2020/3/speech-ed-phumzile-csw64

U.S. Department of Health and Human Services Office of Minority Health (2020, February 14). Heart disease and African Americans. www.minorityhealth.hhs.gov/omh/browse.aspx?lvl=4&lvlid=19

Valasco-Mondragon, E., Jimenez, A., Palladino-Davis, A. G., Davis, D., & Escamilla-Cejudo, J. A. (2016, December 7). Hispanic health in the USA: A scoping review of the literature. *Public Health Review*, *37*, article 31. https://doi.org/10.1186/s40985-016-0043-2

Valeggia, C. R., & Snodgrass, J. J. (2015). Health of Indigenous peoples. *Annual Review of Anthropology*, *44*, 117–135. https://doi.org/10.1146/annurev-anthro-102214-013831

Walter, L. A, & McGregor, A. J. (2020). Sex-and gender-specific observations and implications for COVID-19. *Western Journal of Emergency Medicine: Integrating Emergency Care with Population Health*, *21*(3). http://dx.doi.org/10.5811/westjem.2020.4.47536 https://escholarship.org/uc/item/76f9p924

Welle, D. (2020, May 19). Zero cases: How Pacific islands kept coronavirus at bay. *Taiwan News*. www.taiwannews.com.tw/en/news/3936901

Williams, D. (2016, June 25). What are the causes of poverty? The Borgen Project. Blog post. https://borgenproject.org/what-causes-global-poverty/

Wipfler, P., & Schore, T. (2016). *Listen: Five simple tools to meet your everyday parenting challenges*. Palo Alto, CA: Hand in Hand Parenting.

World Bank (2018, October 17). Nearly half the world lives on less than $5.50 a day. www.worldbank.org/en/news/press-release/2018/10/17/nearly-half-the-world-lives-on-less-than-550-a-day

World Health Organization (WHO) (2010). Pacific Islanders pay heavy price for abandoning traditional diet. Bulletin of the World Health Organization, 88(7), 481–560. www.who.int/bulletin/volumes/88/7/10-010710/en/

World Health Organization (WHO) (2013). Information sheet: Premature death among people with severe mental disorders. www.who.int/mental_health/management/info_sheet.pdf

World Health Organization (WHO) (2017, December 13). World Bank and WHO: Half the world lacks access to essential health services, 100 million still pushed into extreme poverty because of health expenses. News release. www.who.int/news-room/detail/13-12-2017-world-bank-and-who-half-the-world-lacks-access-to-essential-health-services-100-million-still-pushed-into-extreme-poverty-because-of-health-expenses

World Health Organization (WHO) (2018, January). Disability and health. Fact sheet. www.who.int/news-room/fact-sheets/detail/disability-and-health

World Health Organization (WHO) (2019a, April 25). Promoting the health of refugees and migrants 2019–2023: Draft global action plan. https://apps.who.int/gb/ebwha/pdf_files/WHA72/A72_25-en.pdf

World Health Organization (WHO) (2019b). Health and development: Poverty and health. www.who.int/hdp/poverty/en/

World Population Review (2019). *Fertility rate by country 2019*. http://worldpopulationreview.com/countries/total-fertility-rate/

Xu, H., Cupples, L. A., Stokes, A., & Liu, C. (2018). Association of obesity with mortality over 24 years of weight history: Findings from the Framingham Heart Study. *Journal of the American Medical Association*, 1(7), e184587. http://doi:10.1001/jamanetworkopen.2018.4587

Yancy, C. W. (2020, April 15). COVID-19 and African Americans. *Journal of the American Medical Association*, 323(19), 1891–1892. https://doi:10.1001/jama.2020.6548

Young, M. (2019, July 10). What is happening at migrant detention centers: Here is what to know. *Time*. https://time.com/5623148/migrant-detention-centers-conditions/

Zhang, X., Xing, C., Guan, Y., Song, X., Melloy, R., Wang, F., & Jin, X. (2016). Attitudes toward older adults: A matter of cultural values or personal values? *Psychology and Aging*, 31(1), 89–100. http://dx.doi.org/10.1037/pag0000068

INDEX

9 780367 258993